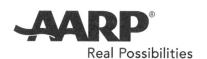

Your Body

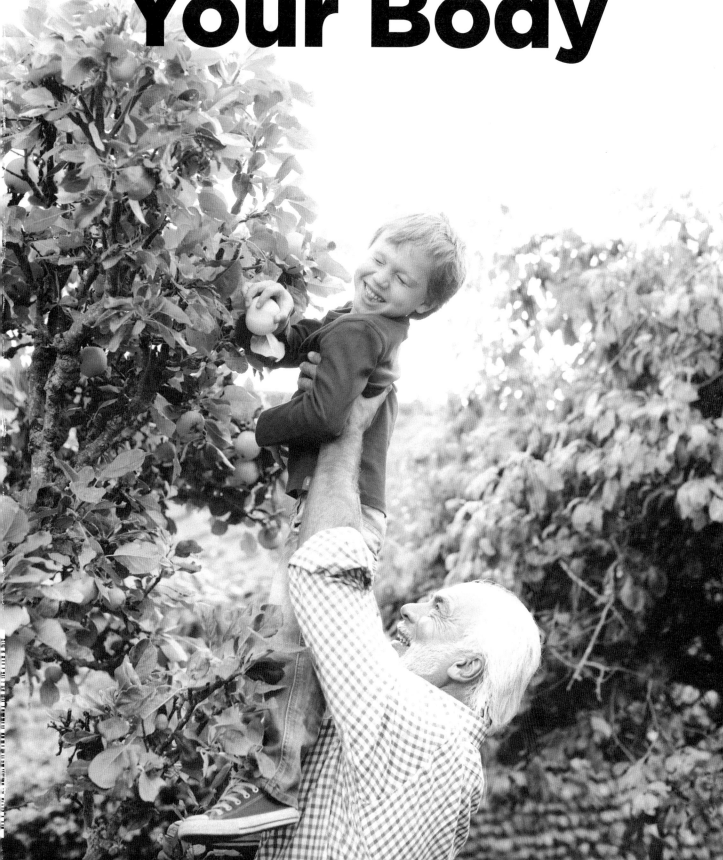

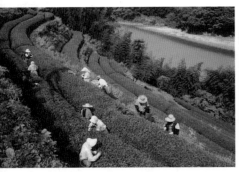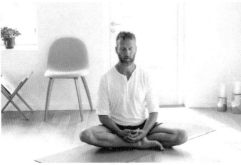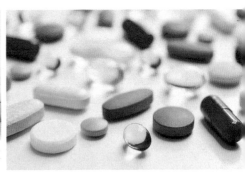

CONTENTS

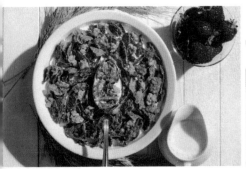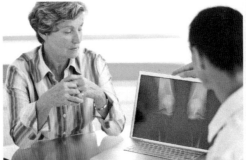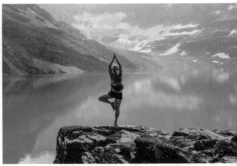

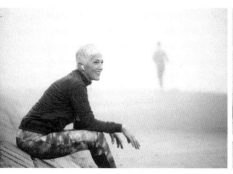
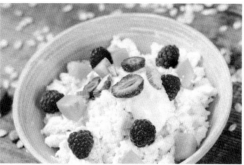
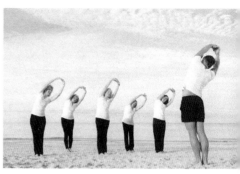

*Some editorial content in this book is reprinted with permission from AARP and individual authors (see page 94).

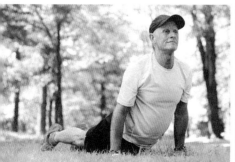
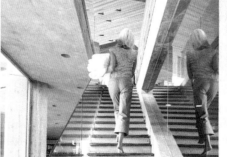
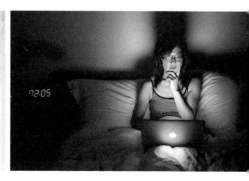

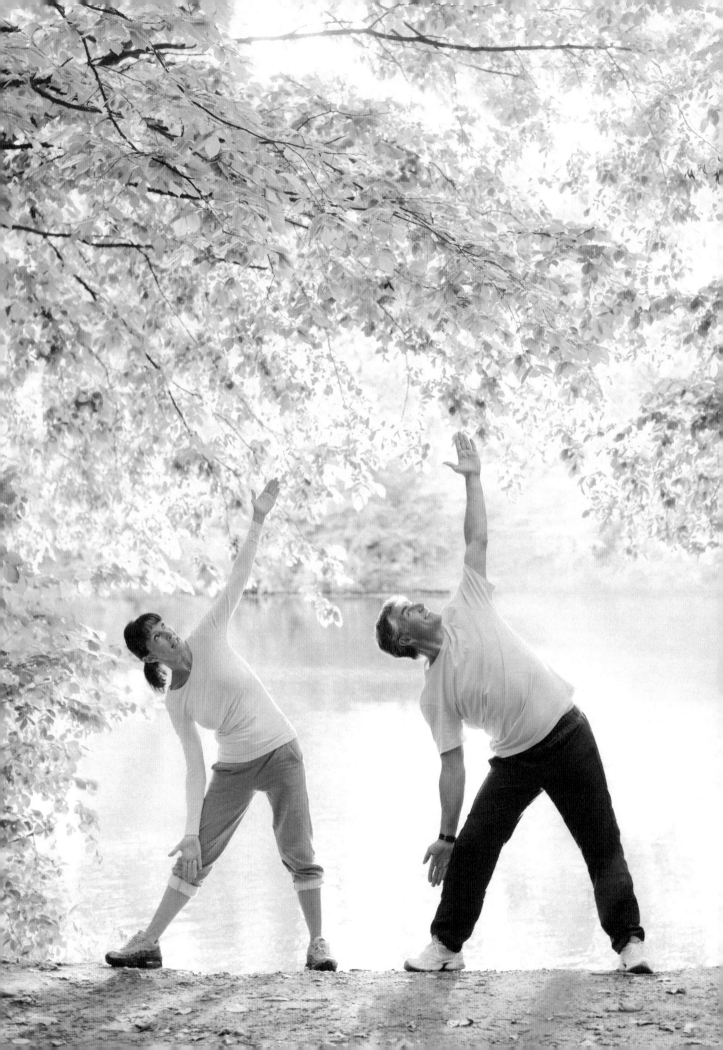

WELCOME TO
YOUR BODY

A message from AARP CEO Jo Ann C. Jenkins

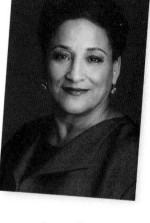

WHEN I WAS A YOUNG PARENT, I recall the guidance and comfort I got from books such as *What to Expect When You're Expecting* and *What to Expect: The Toddler Years.* As we get older and begin experiencing changes in our lives, such solid information, advice and reassurance is harder to come by. I often thought it was too bad that no one had published a book on what to expect at this stage of our lives.

With the publication of *Your Body: Secrets to Living Longer, Better and Healthier,* AARP fills that void. As we grow older, our bodies do change. But for many of us, the line between normal aging and abnormal ailments becomes blurred. Are those achy bones and joints a result of the normal aging process or an indication of a physical problem that can be treated? Are weight gain and reading glasses inevitable? And perhaps more important, even though we want to take more control over our health, we often don't know what to do about it.

Your Body brings together the latest information and insights from AARP's extensive network of experts and resources to help you understand what to expect as you grow older. You'll learn what happens to your body as part of normal aging as well as how factors such as sleep, stress, diet and exercise can help you stay fit and sharp. You'll get the latest research on heart health and bone health, and you'll see why it's important and how to maintain strength and flexibility. You'll also get practical tips on how to sleep better, ways to get the most out of your doctor's visits and which vaccines and surgeries can be beneficial and which ones to avoid. And we'll help guide you through the complex world of medications and alternative health while introducing you to the latest technology to help you take control of your health.

Our goal is not only to help you understand what to expect as you get older, but also to help you discover ways to live longer and better so you can experience the real possibilities that life has in store for you...at every age.

Jo Ann C. Jenkins

Jo Ann C. Jenkins
AARP CEO

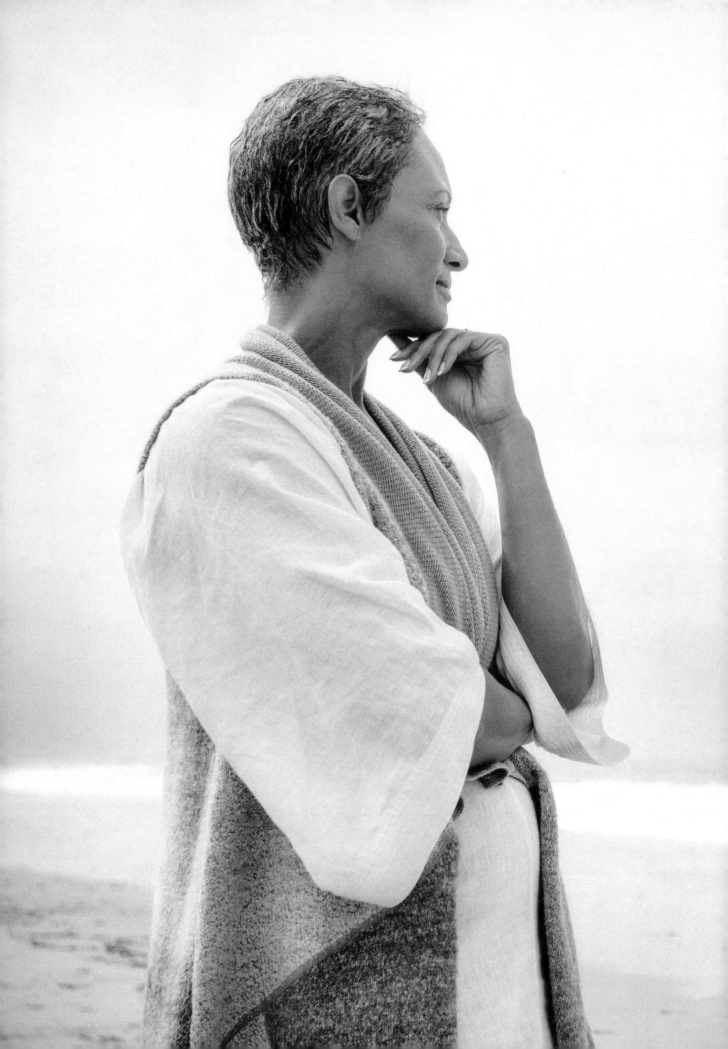

WHAT TO EXPECT IN YOUR 50s, 60s, 70s AND BEYOND

BY BETH HOWARD

YOU KNOW ALL THOSE FEARS you have about aging? Here's a reality check. Aging is not only slow; it's often imperceptible from year to year. "The natural aging process is a relatively minor process until the ninth or tenth decade," says Larry Matson, co-author with Donald M. Vickery, M.D., and Carol Vickery of *Live Young, Think Young, Be Young… At Any Age*. In other words, you won't suddenly wake up a completely different person. It's time to let go of your fears, and embrace what's to come.

So what can you expect through the decades? Better sex. Fewer allergies. More wrinkles but less acne. Each decade offers surprising perks (and a few quirks). Everyone ages differently—and lifestyle plays a major role—but you'll experience both hard-to-notice and impossible-to-miss changes in your physical and mental health. Here are the good, the bad and the various transformations you'll encounter—plus the latest on feeling happy, sexy and pain-free. Check out what's most important to you at your age.

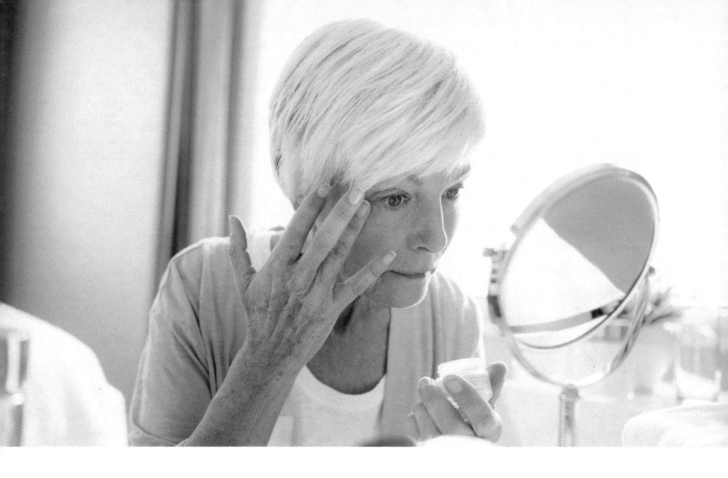

Your Skin

Your skin is likely the first area where you will notice changes. And surprise: some of them are good—like no more pimples.

50s

In your 50s, age spots and skin tags may appear. For the former, consider trying a dermatologist-prescribed hydroquinone product. Skin tags are usually benign. A dermatologist can remove them through freezing, snipping or cauterizing.

The good news? The likelihood of getting an outbreak of acne on the day of your son's wedding is greatly reduced. That's because your skin is getting drier, making blemishes less common. But the loss of muscle, bone and fat under the skin—along with changes in collagen and elastin—makes fine lines and wrinkles more dramatic, especially if you've smoked or sunned significantly. If it bothers you, one remedy is prescription tretinoin products like Retin-A or Renova.

60s

At any age, use SPF 30 sunscreen daily. In your 60s you may develop dilated superficial blood vessels on the cheeks, nose, chin and legs, but if it bothers you, doctors can zap them with a laser that destroys the blood vessels underneath the skin—with no scarring. Another option is a radio-frequency-emitting device, which uses heat to contract collagen and tighten the skin, without injuring the outer epidermis, and platelet rich plasma (PRP) injections that use growth factors in the patient's own blood to pump up volume in the face and neck skin. Also, Botox and injectable fillers can reduce wrinkles. Or consider newcomers Volbella, which targets the fine lines around the lips, and Kybella, which destroys fat pockets under the chin.

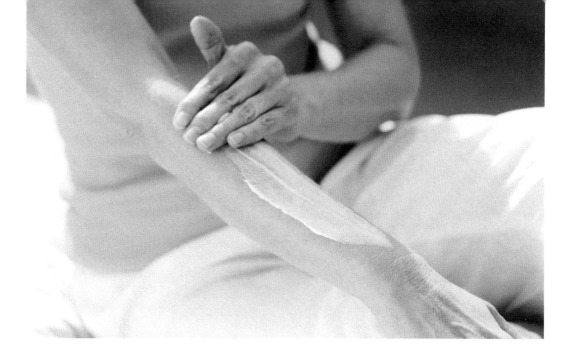

Your skin is drier, so you're less likely to suffer from unsightly breakouts. While some women do experience menopause-related skin issues, they may be treatable with hormone-replacement therapy. You may notice your skin is more fragile, and you may have an increasing number of age spots. Consider using a prescription hydroquinone product. Also, the fine lines and wrinkles that started appearing in your 50s are becoming more dramatic, especially if you smoked or sunned significantly in your younger years. If prescription tretinoin products like Retin-A or Renova don't do the trick, consider injectable fillers.

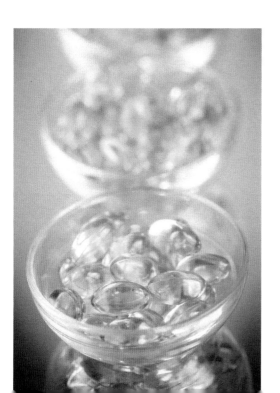

70s

Non-articular cartilage, the type that gives ears and noses their shape, often continues to elongate with age, making these appendages look larger. But look on the bright side: Such cartilage growth may have evolved to enable people to track and funnel sounds and smells as they age.

Drier skin can bring welcome relief for the third of women who were plagued by acne throughout their adulthood. Wrinkles and lines are more plentiful, but so are the options for keeping skin looking bright. Gentle exfoliation and moisturizing are especially important. Pick skin products with antioxidants and glycolic acid, which promote skin thickening and increase collagen production. And apply a broad-spectrum sunscreen 30 every day.

Laser treatments can help with dilated superficial blood vessels, which tend to appear without warning on the cheeks, nose, chin and legs. In your 70s you're likely to notice a big spike in skin tags, as well as excess skin around the neck and jowl lines.

Skin tags are usually benign and can be removed through freezing or cauterizing. If you are bothered by sagging skin under the jaw, consider a skin-tightening radio-frequency treatment or Kybella, a new injectable that dissolves the fat cells.

Your Senses

Lifestyle plays a major role in helping to maintain your sight, hearing and sense of smell.

50s

Floaters, tiny specks of debris in the eye that cast shadows on your retina, can appear in your line of vision. They are typically harmless unless you suddenly see dozens of them.

Your senses of taste, smell and touch remain mostly intact. You'll probably need reading glasses. The cause? As you age, the lenses in your eyes stiffen, making it harder to focus up close. You may become sensitive to glare, and your night vision may decrease, as those same lenses begin to lose clarity. Plus, dry eye becomes more common. Medications like Restasis and Avenova can help with symptoms, as can omega-3 fatty acids like those found in fish.

60s

Lifestyle plays a major role in helping to maintain your senses as you age. So stay away from loud noises, eat a well-balanced diet (which can help ward off some age-related eye disorders) and see a doctor immediately if you notice that your senses of smell or taste diminish significantly. (This may indicate a sinus infection or be a reaction to medication.) Age-related hearing loss becomes more common, primarily as a result of degenerative changes in the inner ear and other structures. About a third of people between ages 65 and 74 have hearing loss, rising to nearly half of those over 75. After age 60, the ability to hear high-frequency tones also diminishes. Swallow your

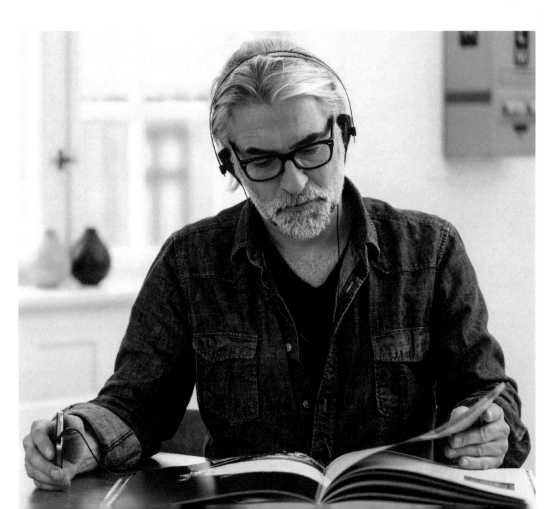

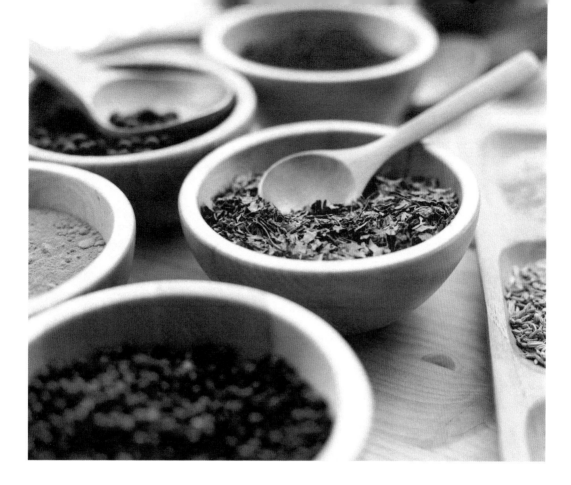

pride and get tested for hearing aids. Plagued by dry eye? Restasis and Avenova can reduce symptoms, and omega-3 fatty acids—found in fish and fish oil supplements—may help tear quality.

You might find it harder to see well in dim light; in general, 60-year-olds need three times as much light to read as 20-year-olds. And after age 60, the risk of macular degeneration increases. Fish oil and a diet rich in antioxidants can help prevent this condition, while vitamin supplements containing vitamin C, vitamin E, lutein, zeaxanthin, zinc oxide and copper have been shown to keep it from progressing.

70s

Have you noticed that vibrant blues and reds appear duller than before? It's just changes in the lenses in your eyes, which have started to yellow and lose clarity with age. If it gets too bad, you may need cataract surgery. About half of people ages 65 to 74 have cataracts; the number rises to more than 70 percent among those 75 or older.

Lifestyle plays a major role in helping to main-

tain your senses as you age. So as in your 60s, stay away from loud noises, eat a well-balanced diet. The not-so-good news: You may have trouble seeing when first entering a very dark or bright area. That's because as you age, your eye muscles slow down, causing your eyes' pupils to react more slowly to changes in light.

After age 70, the ability to see fine details diminishes as well, because there are fewer nerve cells that can effectively transmit visual signals to the brain. If you're plagued by the common issue of dry eye, products including Restasis and Avenova can help.

Finally, some 68 percent of 70-somethings experience some degree of hearing loss. Wearing hearing aids could pay off in the long run, experts say, by helping you stay engaged with others and your environment. After age 70, smell and taste may diminish, reducing the ability to enjoy subtle flavors. Taste buds decrease in number and sensitivity, and nerve endings in the nose may not work as well. Turn up the dial on seasonings. It's an easy fix, and you can experiment with new flavors (but watch the salt!).

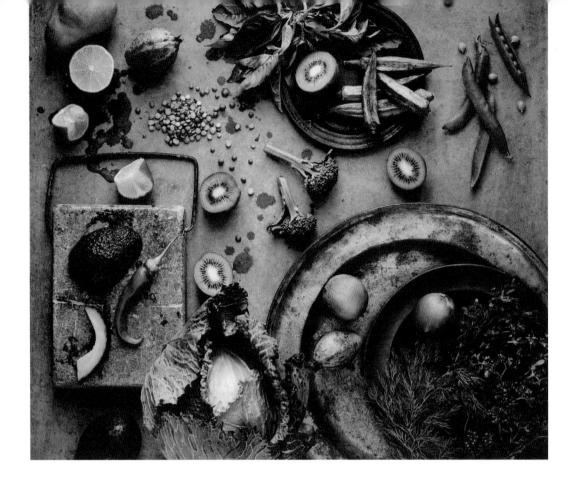

Your Metabolism

Your digestion may change in later years, so be on the lookout for new food sensitivities, and stay active to ward off extra pounds.

50s

After years of guzzling milk with no problem, you may find yourself suffering a dairy hangover—specifically, stomach bloating and discomfort. That's because many people in their 50s produce less lactase, an enzyme that helps digest milk. Even if you're lactose intolerant, you may be able to eat yogurt, which contains active bacterial cultures (known as probiotics) that can help digest lactose.

While metabolism typically slows up to around 5 percent per decade, that doesn't mean you have to gain weight. Just stay active and gradually decrease calories, eating more nutrient-dense foods, including whole grains, fruits and vegetables, low-fat dairy products and fish, says Alice Lichtenstein, director of the Cardiovascular Nutrition Laboratory at the USDA Jean Mayer Human Nutrition Research Center on Aging. "We have fewer 'free' calories for sweets and and soda," she explains. Your stomach empties more slowly, which can increase the risk of reflux. And the slowing of digested material through the large intestine can trigger constipation, says John I. Hughes, M.D., a gastroenterologist with the Kelsey-Seybold Clinic in Houston. The easy fix? Insoluble fiber and water. Adding fiber to your diet may also help protect against colon polyps. By age 50, up to one in four people has had a colon polyp that could lead to cancer, so if you haven't yet scheduled a colonoscopy, make an appointment.

60s

Movement of food through your system slows, increasing the risk for reflux and constipation. Drinking water and adding fiber to your diet can help, plus the roughage may protect against colon polyps. Almost half of those over 60 have colon polyps that may develop into cancer. Be sure to keep up with your regular colonoscopy screenings, especially if previous ones showed adenomas (benign tumors).

Your slowing metabolism—5 percent over this decade—does not doom you to greater girth. Just stay active and cut calories if needed. In your 60s you may secrete less hydrochloric acid, which decreases the availability of vitamin B12, says Lichtenstein. Be alert to symptoms like tiredness, heart palpitations, numbness and tingling. If your doctor agrees, consider more vitamin B12-rich foods or a supplement.

70s

As you age, your ability to produce vitamin D in response to sunlight gradually decreases. Your doctor may recommend a vitamin D supplement—after age 70, you need 800 international units of vitamin D every day, as well as 1,200 milligrams daily of calcium.

Even with a slower metabolic rate, you can maintain a healthy weight in your 70s and beyond. Activity and a few less calories should help. Your body produces less hydrochloric acid in your 70s, which can decrease the vitamin B12 available to your system. Your doctor may advise more vitamin B12-rich foods or a supplement (optimal dose: 2.4 micrograms daily). The sensations of hunger and thirst can also decrease with age, often leading to dehydration and malnutrition. Plan to eat several small meals throughout the day, and consume at least 6 cups of liquid.

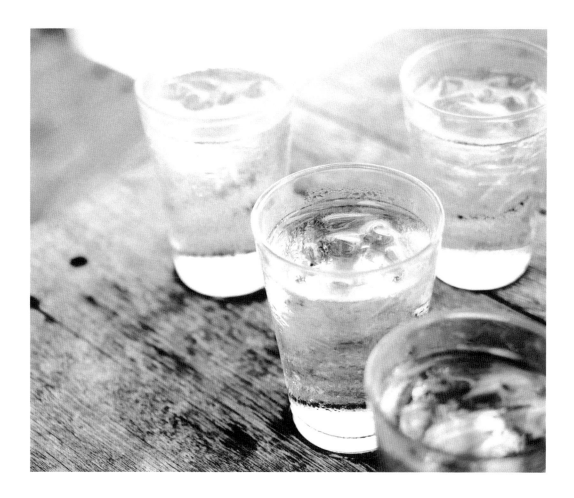

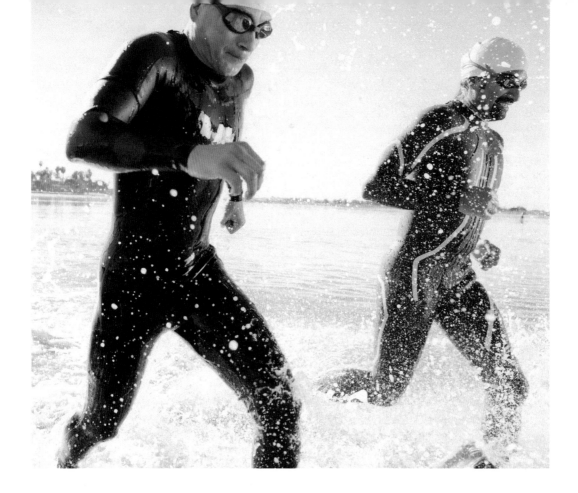

Your Heart

If you're healthy and active, you will likely get a lot more miles out of your ticker. It's never too late to do your part.

50s

Have you noticed a skipped beat or a racing heart? It could be atrial fibrillation, a type of heart arrhythmia that becomes more common with age. Since it can increase the risk of stroke, mention it to your doctor. You should also tell him or her if you're experiencing unusual fatigue, weakness or dizziness when exercising.

Your heart's walls are getting thicker and its valves are stiffer. Also, many people in their 50s will start to develop the first signs of heart disease. Thanks to new treatments and the mitigation of risk factors like high cholesterol, the death rate from heart disease dropped about 39 percent from 2001 to 2011, according to the American Heart Association.

60s

A skipped beat or a racing heart could be atrial fibrillation, a type of heart arrhythmia that becomes more common with age. Since it can increase the risk of stroke, mention it to your doctor.

An older heart can pump about the same volume of blood with each beat as a younger one can. Heart disease accounts for around 30 percent of all deaths among men and women age 65 and over. But thanks to advances in the treatment of this disease, the death rate from heart disease dropped. One way to improve your odds? Keep moving. The Centers for Disease Control and Prevention recommends 150 minutes of moderately intense activity a week to reduce the risk of heart disease and stroke.

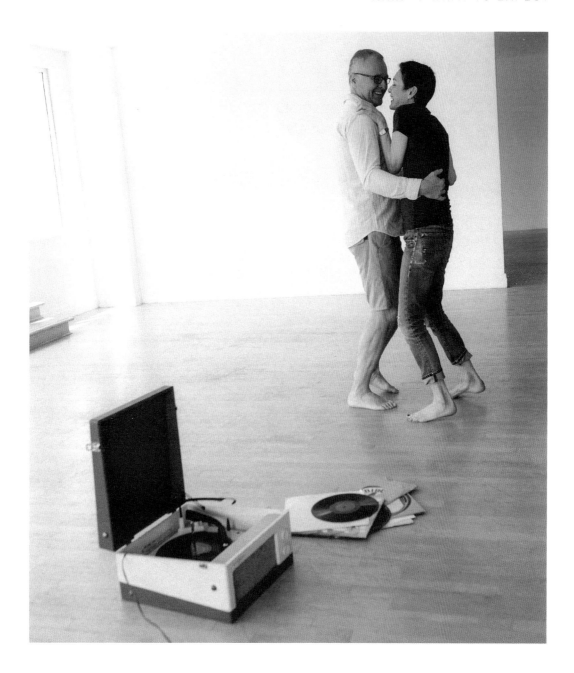

70s

You are more likely than ever to experience the sudden racing of the heart or skipped beats, the telltale signs of a heart rhythm problem like atrial fibrillation, which increases the risk of stroke. Let your doctor know if you notice it or if you're experiencing unusual fatigue, weakness when exercising or dizziness.

Your ticker still pumps the same amount of blood per beat as it did when you were younger.

Your heart's walls naturally thicken with age, and the heart valves, which propel blood through its chambers, are less pliable.

One sure way to improve your heart health? Keep moving. Research shows that women and men age 70-plus who spent as little as a half hour a day on activities like walking and dancing had a 20 to 40 percent lower risk of dying from heart disease than those who reported no activity. Staying active is one of the best forms of preventive medicine.

Your Bones and Joints

If you've been active, your bones, joints and muscles have a better chance of staying in good shape. And if you've been sedentary, get moving.

50s

Your joints may snap, crackle and pop, but those noises are usually harmless unless the joints are also painful and swollen. Those sounds may be ligaments tightening around a moving joint, a tendon snapping over a joint or nitrogen bubbles "popping" in the fluid inside a joint. But talk to your doctor if you have pain, swelling or numbness. Aging and inactivity can lead to achy joints

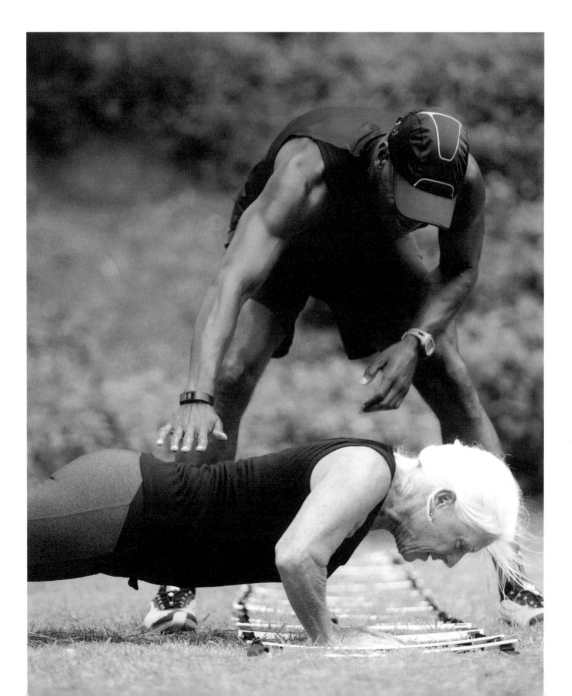

because of the wearing down of cartilage, the loss of lubricating joint fluid and weaker muscles. Maintain a healthy weight, and do strength training.

60s

Those popping and cracking noises coming from your joints may sound scary, but unless they're also painful and swollen, don't worry.

Had an active life up until now? Your bones, joints and muscles will continue to serve you well in your 60s. If you've been sedentary, you may develop painful, swollen joints, thanks to the loss of cartilage, lubricating joint fluid and muscle strength. Keep a normal weight and do weight-bearing exercises, which stimulate the bones to grow stronger and denser. Also, talk to your doctor about vitamin D and calcium supplements. The recommended dose of vitamin D is 600 international units a day; women in their 60s need about 1,200 milligrams of calcium a day.

70s

Although worn joints may benefit from anti-inflammatory drugs and activity, surgery may become necessary as cartilage loss begins to accelerate. Regenerative techniques such as platelet-rich plasma and autologous (self) stem cell injections may also help.

You can maintain muscle strength through activity. About one in four women in their 70s—and more than a third of women in their 80s—have osteoporosis in their hip or spine, which greatly increases the risk of fractures. Studies show strength training can build muscle, which can take force off the joints, plus stimulate the bones to grow stronger and denser.

Although worn joints may benefit from anti-inflammatory drugs and activity, surgery may become necessary as cartilage loss begins to accelerate. Regenerative techniques such as platelet-rich plasma and autologous (self) stem cell injections may also help, according to Nathan Wei, M.D., a rheumatologist in Frederick, Maryland.

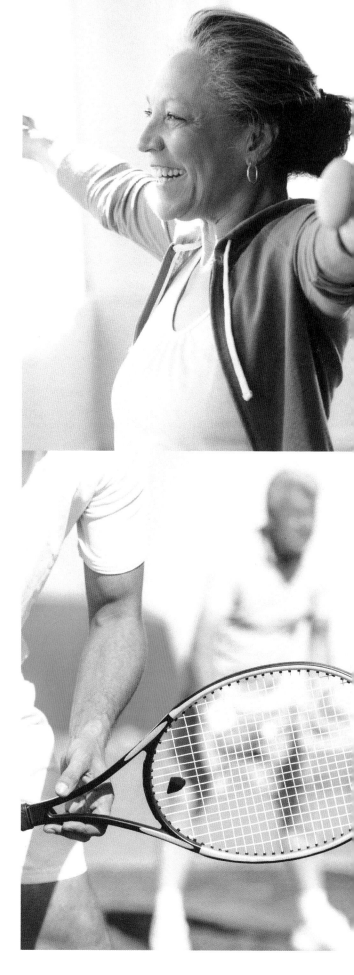

Your Sex Life

Sex for men and women can be as fulfilling as it was in your younger years—or even better. Numerous remedies are available to treat erectile dysfunction and the side effects of menopause.

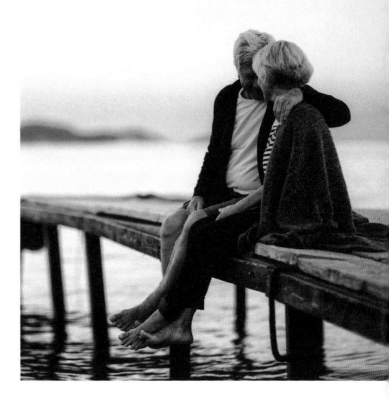

50s

Rates of erectile dysfunction (ED) increase with age; among men with the condition, 26 percent first experienced symptoms in their 50s. Research shows that the Mediterranean diet—rich in fish, nuts, vegetables and olive oil—helps, particularly for men at risk of cardiovascular disease. Lifestyle changes like exercising and not lighting up can also make a difference.

Sex after 50 can be better than it was during the child-raising years: You've got more time and fewer distractions, and you're not exhausted from day-to-day child-care issues. Sex-related hormones—estrogen and progesterone in women, testosterone in men—are declining in your 50s, although these dips are less likely to diminish your sex life than are bad habits like smoking and a sedentary lifestyle.

60s

Men may experience ED; in one study of those with ED, 40 percent first noticed symptoms in their 60s. Try kicking the habit, working out and eating well to keep your sex life strong.

Sex in your 60s can be hotter than ever: Getting older often means becoming more comfortable in your own skin. In fact, sexual satisfaction among women rises with age, a University of California, San Diego School of Medicine–led study found. In that study, two-thirds of sexually active women (with a median age of 67) were moderately or very satisfied with their sex lives. An active lifestyle can drive it up further. Waning estrogen and progesterone in women and dwindling testosterone in men can put a damper on sex. Vaginal dryness may become more noticeable, but over-the-counter lubricants are effective, as are prescription creams and tablets.

70s

By 70, between 40 and 60 percent of men will experience symptoms of ED. But staying active, not smoking and eating well can keep the problem at bay. Devices, implants and pharmaceutical fixes can also help sidestep it.

Research shows that 70-year-old men and women were much more likely to be sexually active, to report being in a happy relationship and to have a positive attitude toward sex than people that age who were polled in the 1970s. Some 44 percent of women ages 68 to 80 report being very satisfied with their sex lives, compared with just 30 percent of women 55 to 68 years old. Vaginal discomfort increases as sex hormones dip in women. Over-the-counter lubricants as well as estrogen creams and tablets can mitigate the problem.

Your Immune System

Your response to vaccines decreases with age, leaving you even more vulnerable to illnesses like flu and pneumonia. Here's how to keep strong.

50s

You may be able to boost the effectiveness of your vaccines by getting enough sleep: Research shows that those who slept less than six hours a night produced fewer antibodies after receiving a vaccine.

Allergies, which result from an overreactive immune system, may become less severe, primarily because your immune system isn't as sensitive, says James Stankiewicz, M.D., Medical Director of Audiology and ENT at Loyola University Medical Center in Maywood, Ill. A less aggressive immune response means you're more susceptible to getting sick. Protect yourself by shedding excess pounds, eating well and exercising.

60s

After 65 you're eligible to get a higher-dose flu vaccine. In your 60s you'll also need vaccines against shingles and pneumococcal disease, as these conditions mostly strike after age 60.

Allergies are probably a thing of the past, because your immune system isn't as sensitive.

A weaker immune system can lead to more illness. And chronic inflammation can make you even more vulnerable. This condition is linked to heart disease, diabetes and arthritis, so it's important to lose excess weight, consume a healthy diet and exercise.

70s

Ask your doctor if the higher-dose flu vaccine, which creates a stronger immune response, is right for you. Research also suggests you can boost the effectiveness of your vaccines by getting at least seven hours of sleep a night. Plus, older people who eat at least five servings of fruits and vegetables daily mount a better response to pneumonia vaccine than those who skimp. Scientists are also investigating an agent called spermidine that may enhance the response to vaccines.

Thanks to a less robust immune response, you may be more likely to fall ill. Dropping unhealthy pounds, eating a good diet and exercising regularly can help by calming chronic inflammation, the culprit behind many chronic conditions, including heart disease, diabetes and arthritis.

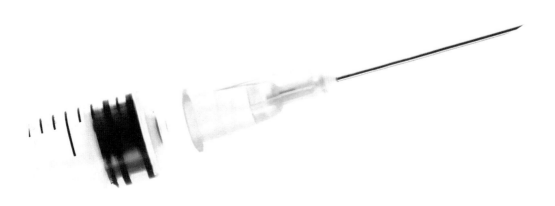

Your Bladder

If you're generally healthy, your urological system likely works just about as well as it did when you were younger. Getting older poses a few additional challenges, but most are manageable.

50s

Benign prostatic hyperplasia, or symptoms of an enlarged prostate gland, affects about 50 percent of men between the ages of 51 and 60 and up to 90 percent of men older than 80. Symptoms include difficulty urinating, though medications can help.

In their 50s, 50 percent of men and women experience occasional nocturia, getting up twice a night (or more) to urinate. Try decreasing fluids after 6 p.m. and avoiding caffeinated beverages. If you're on diuretics for high blood pressure, speak to your doctor about taking your pill in the morning. Stress incontinence—urine loss when coughing or sneezing—affects more than half of all women over 50 at some point. You can reduce incontinence symptoms through bladder training, medications and Kegel exercises. If these measures don't work, ask about platelet-rich plasma (PRP) injections, which help shore up the urethra and surrounding areas.

60s

Find yourself running to the bathroom all the time? You may have overactive bladder, a condition caused by bladder muscles that contract sporadically. Many people write it off as just another symptom of aging, but you don't have to live with it: Kegels, meds, bladder training and Botox injections may help.

If you're generally healthy, your urological system likely works about as well as when you were younger. And an array of therapies can help when problems crop up. Gotta go once during the night? Not to worry; that's normal during this decade.

70s

Gotta go during the night? If you're generally healthy, your urological system likely functions pretty well. And an array of therapies can help when problems crop up. Bladder tissue contracts and expands less efficiently as you get older, often leading to overactive bladder, incontinence and infection.

About 60 percent of women in their 70s will experience some type of urinary incontinence. Ask your doctor about bladder training, medications and pelvic floor exercises (Kegels), or newer methods, such as Botox injections (which help to reduce bladder contractions) and platelet-rich plasma (PRP) injections (which help shore up the urethra and surrounding areas). An enlarged prostate gland, called benign prostatic hyperplasia (BPH), may affect up to 90 percent of men over 70, producing symptoms such as a weak urine flow or difficulty urinating, but medications—including the ED drug Cialis—are often helpful.

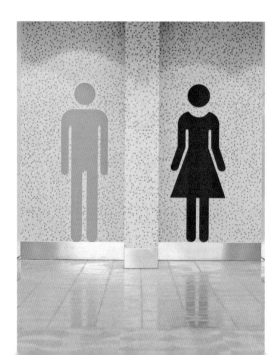

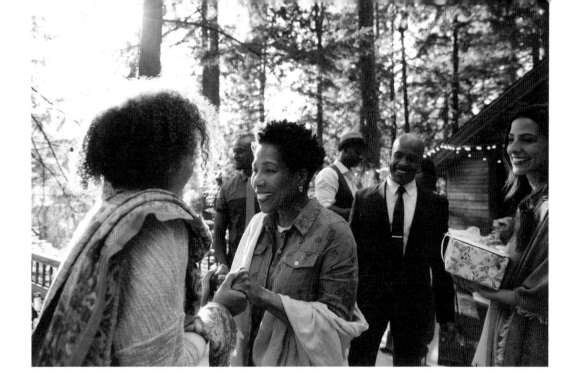

Your Mental Health

Your 50s, 60s and 70s may just be your happiest decades ever.

50s

Mental illness is a serious issue, so if you are concerned, seek professional help. But there is good news. The ability to regulate one's emotions improves as you get older. That means situations that might once have tied you up in knots no longer bother you as much.

In fact, as we age, we get happier. An AARP survey showed that from your early 50s on, happiness rises significantly over time. One explanation for the trend: years of experience. You know that bad times pass—and good ones, which makes them more precious. New research also suggests that you experience greater trust at this point in life. That may help you to derive more satisfaction from social relationships, boosting happiness.

60s

AARP research shows that from your early 50s on, happiness increases. A new study from Buffalo and Northwestern universities also points to the role of trust, which grows as you age. It allows people to get more support and comfort from friends and family, improving their sense of well-being.

70s

Social networks may shrink, but contentment soars. An AARP survey showed that of all the decades surveyed, the 70s tend to be some of the happiest years of your life. There are several reasons for the trend. "As you get older, you know that bad times are going to pass," says Laura Carstensen, Ph.D., director of the Stanford Center on Longevity. "You also know that good times will pass, which makes those good times even more precious." Another factor: a greater sense of trust, which lets people derive more from their social relationships, thus enhancing their happiness. Be sure to keep up social ties, which are important to facing the future with resilience. And if you are concerned about your mental health, seek professional help. ■

STRENGTH AND FLEXIBILITY

AS WE GET OLDER, INCREASING and maintaining our strength and flexibility becomes even more important, and we gain even more benefits from these practices. While it is critical to our overall health that we remain active and get our hearts pumping several times a week, it is just as essential to build our muscles and stretch them out. These complementary activities help to keep our bodies truly well-rounded.

Strength training is not about being able to lift heavy weights (although if you're so inclined, it's a wonderful practice). We need to build up our muscle strength so that we can go about our daily lives without strain, pain or too much assistance. In this section you won't find any admonitions about getting to the gym or working on machines; instead, we provide a step-by-step plan for doing 11 exercises that will systematically work your entire body. You can do these moves next to your bed first thing in the morning, when you're catching up on your favorite show, or while you're waiting in line—they work anywhere, at any time.

Part of being strong is having energy, and we provide information that covers the best choices for keeping you active and lively, from what to choose for breakfast to how long to nap, to whether you're better off making a list of what needs to be done or what you're grateful for (hint: being productive is not always the fastest road to feeling energized).

The flip side of having strong muscles is keeping them loose and limber. Time can contribute to decreased flexibility and tightness, and stretching counteracts this tendency and can help prevent injury. And the best part about stretching? It feels so good.

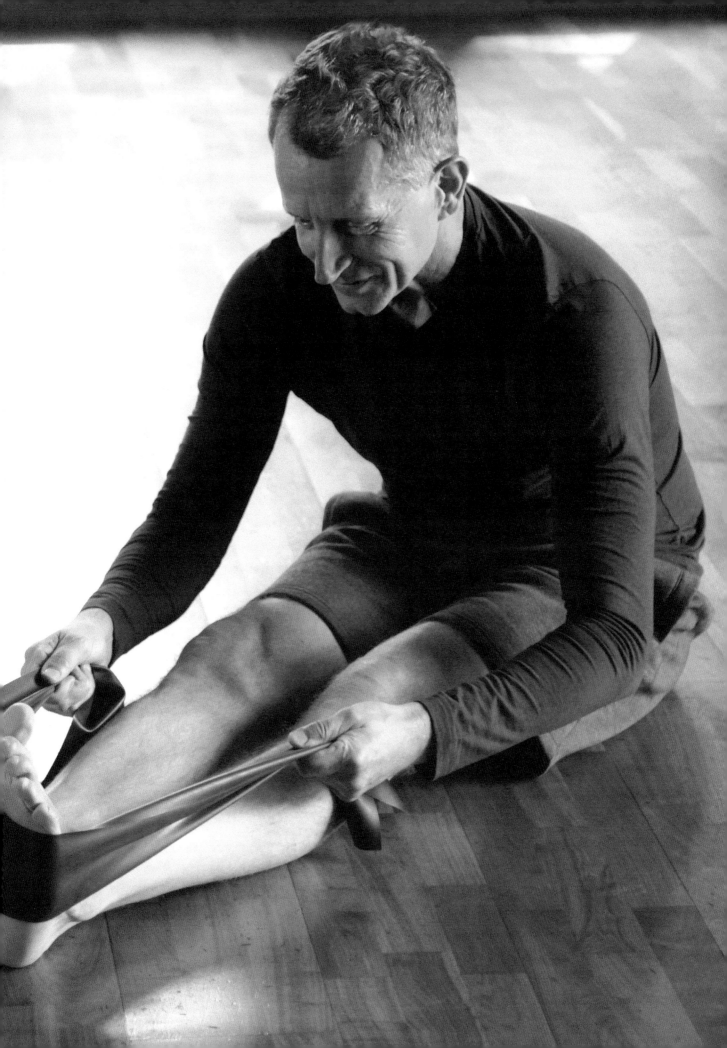

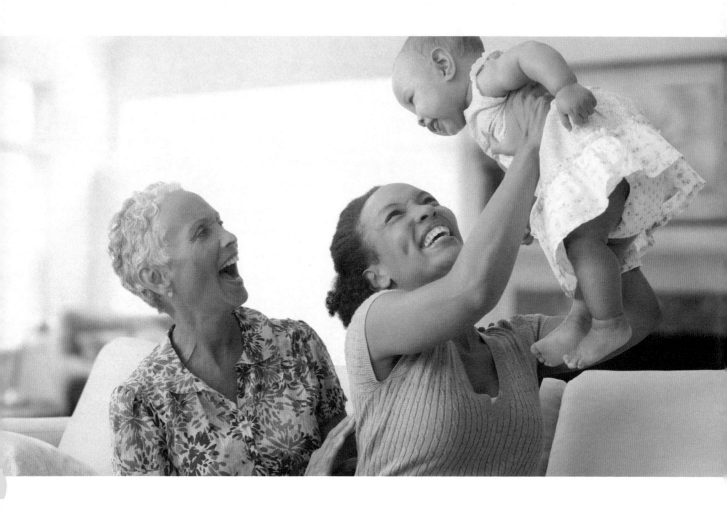

MOVES TO MAKE YOU HEALTHIER AND STRONGER

Strength training exercises that can help you in your daily activities, from vacuuming your home to playing with the grandkids

BY BETH HOWARD

EVER STRAIN YOUR BACK WHILE carrying laundry? Or find yourself so sore from gardening that you can't stand straight the next day? Some everyday movements require groups of muscles to work together in harmony, and unless you're exercising all of them, you're likely to end up with back or leg pain. For best results, do each set of exercises three times a week.

These exercises are designed to be done in the home, or anywhere with a level surface where you have a bit of space. You need only sturdy shoes and a set of light weights. If you don't have weights, use canned goods or water bottles (fill with water slowly and stop when you get to a weight that feels good). Make sure your "weights" are identical and fit comfortably in your hands.

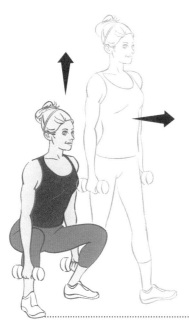

1. TAKING IN GROCERIES

Carrying heavy groceries can strain your neck, shoulders and lower back.

The fix: Squat, lift and carry

1. Stand with your feet hip-width apart and with small weights on each side of you on the floor.
2. Bend your knees and pick up a weight in each hand. Straighten and walk 10 to 30 paces, then set down the weights.
3. Turn around, pick up the weights and walk back. Repeat 3 times.

2. LOADING AND UNLOADING THE DISHWASHER

All that bending and lifting can torque your lower back unless your hips are flexible.

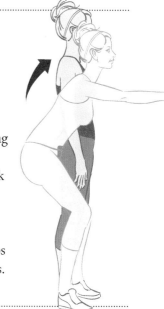

The fix: Hip hinge

1. Start with your feet hip-width apart, your knees slightly bent, neck long and shoulder blades tucked gently down and in, arms by your sides.
2. Move your hips backward and bend your knees, still keeping your back long and straight. Your torso should lean forward from your hips.
3. Slowly extend your arms straight in front of you. Go only as far as you can while maintaining proper posture.
4. Pause, then slowly rise, straightening your knees and moving your hips and arms back to the starting position. Do 3 sets of 10 to 15 repetitions.

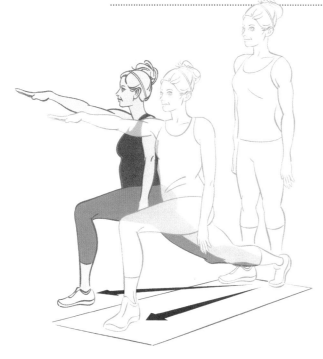

3. VACUUMING

Running a vacuum cleaner can tire your back and core as you lunge, bend and pivot to clean hard-to-reach places.

The fix: Lunge and reach

1. Start with your feet hip-width apart and your knees slightly bent.
2. Step forward with your left leg, bending the left and right knees while reaching forward with your right hand.
3. Rise out of the lunge, coming back to the starting position.
4. Now do a diagonal lunge: Step out with your left leg to the left side while reaching out with your right arm.
5. Repeat on the other side, first stepping forward with your right leg, then rising and lunging out to the right. Do 3 sets of 10 to 15 repetitions on each side.

4. GETTING UP OFF THE FLOOR

Picking yourself up off the floor involves multiple muscles and can be difficult if your upper body is weak.

The fix: Stationary diagonal lunge

1. Stand near a railing, keeping a hand on it for stability.
2. Step to the left, then bend both knees. Rise, switch sides and repeat. Do 3 sets of 10 to 15 repetitions.

The fix: Modified push-up

1. Start in an all-fours position on a mat or soft carpet, hands in front of your shoulders, knees on the floor.
2. Slowly lower your torso toward the floor as far as you can, then lift up, extending your elbows as you go. Do 3 sets of 5 to 15 repetitions.

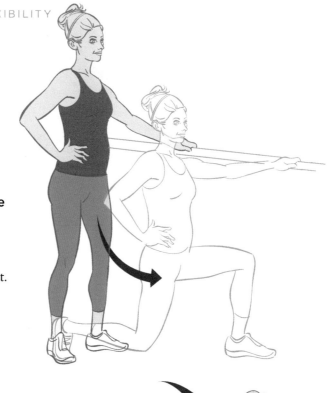

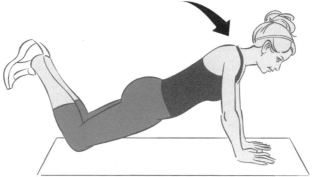

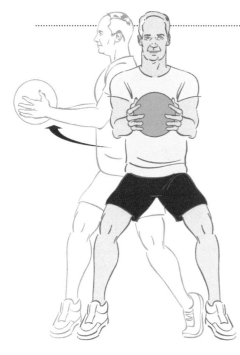

5. PUTTING A CHILD INTO A CAR SEAT

Bending over with a heavy object (a child) requires strong back and arm muscles. You'll also need to work on building a strong core.

The fix: Squat, lift and twist

1. Start with your feet hip-width apart. While holding a medicine ball (or other weight) in both hands, slowly bend your knees and move your hips backward into a squat.
2. Twist gently to the left, then return to the starting position.
3. Repeat, twisting your torso to the right. Do 2 to 3 sets of 5 to 10 repetitions.

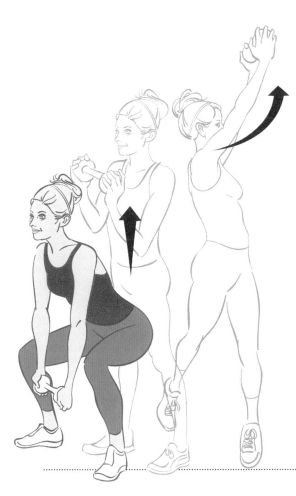

6. PUTTING LUGGAGE INTO THE OVERHEAD BIN

Lifting heavy suitcases over your head can tax your back, shoulders, chest and obliques—the muscles that run down the sides of your torso.

The fix: Squat, press and twist

1. Start with your feet hip-width apart and your knees bent.
2. Slowly bend your knees into a mini-squat position, moving your hips backward slightly.
3. Rise out of the squat while lifting a small weight to chest level.
4. Raise the object over your head while twisting gently to the left, then twist back to center and lower the object.
5. Repeat, raising the object to the right side. Do 2 to 3 sets of 5 reps on each side.

7. STAIR CLIMBING

Whether you're touring Rome or hiking in Yellowstone, you'll likely be doing more walking and stair climbing than you would on a normal day.

The fix: Step-up

1. Start with a step stool between 6 and 12 inches high.
2. Step up with your right leg, with your left leg following. Then step down.
3. Next, step up with your left leg first. Do 2 to 3 sets of 5 step-ups on each side.

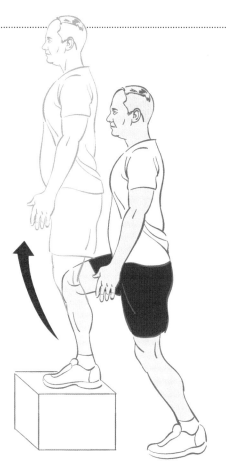

8. PICKING UP TOYS OFF THE FLOOR

If your grandkids are over, there's a good chance the floor is littered with toys. Collect them without pulling a muscle by strengthening the muscles in your back and legs.

The fix: Sumo squat

1. Start with your feet hip-width apart, your toes pointing out slightly and your knees slightly bent.
2. Lower gently into a squat, moving your hips down and back, and bending your torso forward slightly.
3. While in the squatting position, move your right hand toward your left toes, as if picking up an imaginary object.
4. Push up firmly, through your heels and mid-feet, out of the squat.
5. Repeat on the other side, moving your left hand toward your right toes. Do 3 sets of 10 to 15 repetitions, 3 days a week.

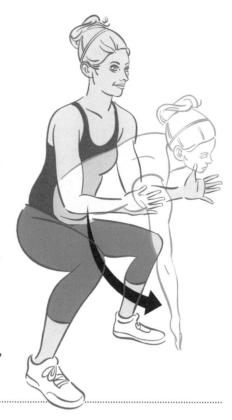

9. GARDENING

Planting, digging and weeding can tax your core, arms and legs. This simple exercise targets them all, making gardening fun—and pain free.

The fix: Bird dog

1. Start from an all-fours position, with your back flat, a neutral pelvis and your eyes looking down.
2. Slowly extend your right arm forward to shoulder height and lift your left leg back and up to hip height.
3. Pause, then slowly lower your arm and leg to the starting position.
4. Repeat on the other side. Do 3 sets of 10 to 15 repetitions, 3 days a week.

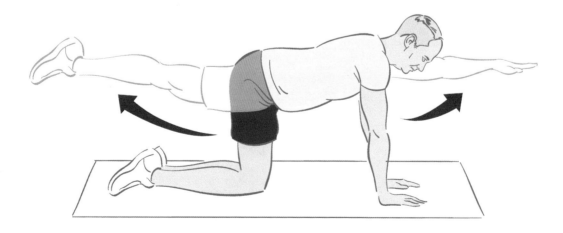

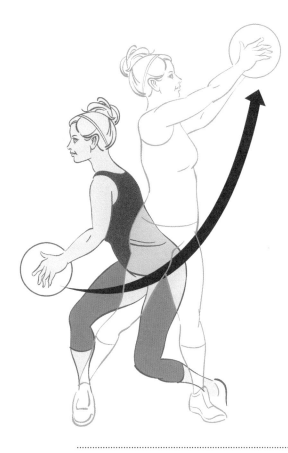

10. SPORTS MOVES

Many sports—from tennis to golf to kayaking—rely on your ability to rotate your torso effectively. This move features a mid-body twist that engages muscles along the entire midsection.

The fix: Hay baler with mini squat

1. Start with your feet hip-width apart, your weight in your mid-feet and heels.
2. Holding a weighted object (such as a medicine ball) beside your left hip, inhale as you slowly bend your knees and move your hips backward into a mini squat.
3. Press evenly into your heels and mid-feet as you rise from the squat, twisting your torso from left to right, while moving the object diagonally across your body and above your right shoulder.
4. Switch sides and repeat. Do 2 to 3 sets of 5 repetitions, 3 days a week.

11. SEX

Inflexible hip joints, upper-body weakness and muscle imbalances can put a damper on your sex life. These two exercises can build and even boost your sexual fitness.

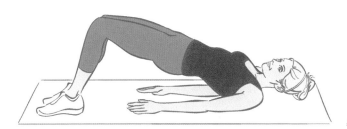

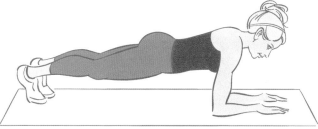

The fix: Bridge

1. Lie flat on your back with both knees bent, arms by your sides.
2. Press your weight evenly into both feet, and slowly raise your lower, middle and then upper back off the floor.
3. Pause when your thighs, hips and chest are in one parallel plane. Keep your neck long to avoid putting pressure on it.
4. Slowly lower your upper, middle and lower back to the starting position. Do 3 sets of 10 to 15 repetitions, 3 days a week.

The fix: Plank

1. Lie facedown on a mat or soft carpet. Align your elbows under your shoulders.
2. Press your forearms and toes into the floor and raise your body off it. Keep your spine in alignment and your lower back flat throughout the exercise.
3. Hold your body in the plank position for 10 to 20 seconds, breathing normally, then slowly lower and rest. Do 3 sets of planks, 3 days a week. ■

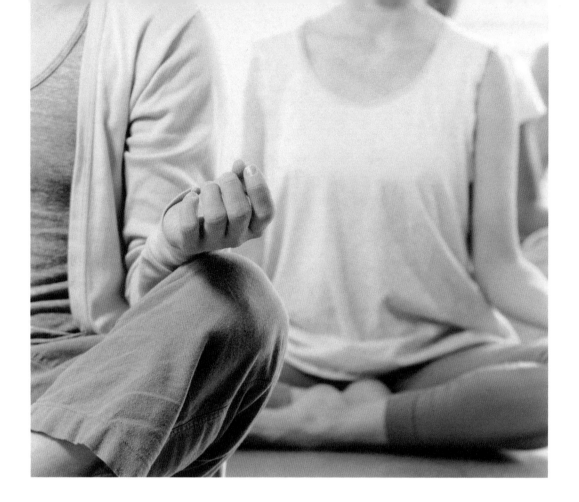

GET MORE ENERGY

Discover new ways to boost everyday vigor

BY SARI HARRAR

LIFE SPARKLES WHEN YOU'RE energized. Getting through a day of work or errands is a cinch, and having leftover zip for fun with family and friends is what life is really all about.

But energy—the human kind—seems to be in short supply these days. Only 1 in 7 Americans, or just 15 percent, say they wake up feeling rested. And just as having energy can bolster most aspects of your life, lacking energy can negatively affect your health and well-being. Fatigue can squelch good moods, increase risk for depression and mess with your weight, sex life and productivity at work. Take this quiz to test your knowledge on how to boost your stamina, and to discover simple, proven ways to turn up your energy dial, each and every day.

Q Energy drink or water?
A WATER. Both brain and muscle cells need water for optimal performance. Energy drinks contain loads of extra sodium, caffeine and other stimulants (not to mention calories from simple sugars) that you just don't need; downing just one can boost blood pressure 6 percent.

Q Long nap or short nap?
A SHORT. Cuddle on the couch, close your office door or set your car seat on recline (while parked, obviously) for a power snooze. A quick nap can boost performance 34 percent without the after-nap grogginess that researchers call sleep inertia. Longer naps drop you into slow-wave sleep, leaving you disoriented and sleepy for longer when you do wake up.

Q Whole grain cereal with milk or pancakes with syrup?

A WHOLE GRAIN CEREAL WITH MILK. Sure, you'll feel revved up when those pancakes first hit your bloodstream. But the energy in simple sugars is released very quickly—in about 20 to 30 minutes—and can leave you at a lower energy level than when you started. Go with whole grains and protein instead.

Q Moderate- or low-intensity exercise?

A LOW-INTENSITY. Tired? Low-intensity exercise (the pace of an easy walk) could pep you up. When 24 inactive, always-fatigued people started brand-new workouts for a University of Georgia study, the turtles won. Volunteers pedaled exercise bikes at low or moderate intensity for 20 minutes three times a week; a third group didn't exert themselves at all. After six weeks, all exercisers felt 20 percent more energetic—but the low-intensity group felt less fatigued by the workouts than the moderate-intensity group did.

Q Sit or stand while working?

A STAND. Standing up while working increases productivity 10 to 46 percent, studies have shown. Increased blood circulation or the release of mood-boosting hormones may explain why standing gives energy a boost. Stanford University researchers think it may be the reason people in one study came up with more than twice as many creative thoughts while walking as they did while sitting.

Q Tea or coffee?

A TEA. Too tired for your Zumba class? Try sipping some green or black tea instead of a cup of joe. Sure, the heftier caffeine dose in the coffee will rev you up, but it can also leave you jittery, interfere with sleep tonight (so you feel more tired tomorrow) and even put you on a roller coaster of caffeine highs and withdrawals that'll leave you hankering for more. By contrast, tea contains a lower dose of caffeine than coffee but can decrease tiredness by 14 percent.

Q Turkey burger or grilled-steak salad?

A STEAK SALAD. A turkey burger can be surprisingly high in fat, while a grilled-steak salad with a splash of vinaigrette can have much less. Keeping fat low can keep energy high. A high-fat lunch can torpedo energy by as much as 20 percent more than a low-fat meal, according to a British study. Instead, pair lean protein with fruit, veggies and whole grains for lasting zing.

Q Meditation or happy hour?

A MEDITATION. More than half of Americans who experience stress say it tires them out. But joining friends or coworkers at a happy hour can leave you feeling more fatigued, due to the sedative effects of alcohol (and for some, the hubbub of a loud, full bar). Learning a variety of mindfulness techniques—to use while walking, eating or sitting quietly—and practicing just five to 20 minutes a day improved energy by 28 percent in people with sleep problems in one University of Southern California study.

Q Review your to-do list or count your blessings?

A COUNT YOUR BLESSINGS. Sure, it's important to check things off your to-do list—and enjoy your accomplishments. But spending time feeling gratitude and appreciation for the blessings in your life can help you feel more energetic.

Q Chewing gum, sunshine or a random act of kindness?

A ALL OF THE ABOVE. Sounds crazy, but chomping on gum enhanced mental alertness and memory by about 30 percent—for about 15 to 20 minutes. Experts suspect that chewing stimulates blood flow to the brain. Sitting by a sunny window for 30 minutes increased alertness in one Japanese study. And learning something new or focusing on what brings most joy in your job counted among the most revitalizing strategies in a recent study. Biggest energy drain: complaining. ■

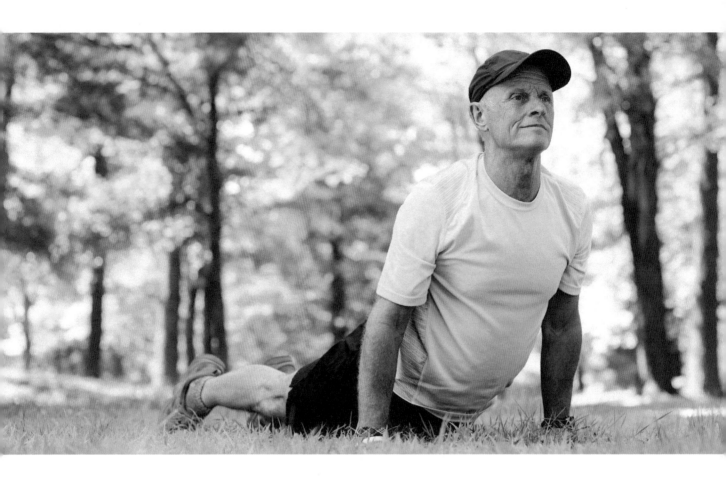

INCREASE YOUR FLEXIBILITY

If you don't use it, you'll lose it

I F YOU'RE A DOG OR CAT OWNER, you've probably noticed how often your pet likes to stretch. Stretching feels good, especially after lying around all day. Or, as is more often the case with humans, sitting around all day. But unlike our furry friends, we're not as likely to get up and stretch our bodies after long bouts of inactivity, even though our bodies would like nothing more. From sitting all day at a desk or computer, we usually move on to a seat in a car, bus or train, and then home to more seated activity—eating, reading, watching television shows, paying bills, answering email.

With 28 percent of people over the age of 50 leading an inactive life, is there any wonder that we see more health problems related to joints and muscles that rebel by becoming stiff, sore and even painful? Aging, too, contributes to tight muscles and poor flexibility because, as we age, muscles tend to become less elastic and tissues around the joints thicken. That hampers movement. In fact, you can lose 10 percent of your flexibility every 10 years if you do nothing.

> Stay Loose

Stretching helps keep your muscles loose, which improves your flexibility. Regular stretching can make you more mobile, making it easier to bend down, as well as reach for things in cupboards, says Jay Blahnik, director of fitness for health technologies at Apple and author of the book *Full-Body Flexibility*. "It's like a reward that you can feel every day." There are other rewards too. Staying flexible can help you:

> Improve and maintain your range of motion, which improves balance
> Prevent falls
> Relieve chronic pain
> Reduce tension and stress
> Improve circulation and concentration
> Boost your energy
> Improve your posture

> Prevent Injuries

Recommendations to stretch or not to stretch are full of misconceptions and conflicting research. There is limited evidence to sort out these issues. Stretching has been promoted for years as an essential part of fitness programs to decrease the risk of injury, prevent soreness and improve performance. But what does the evidence say? Current research suggests that stretching can decrease pain and soreness after exercise. And recently, some evidence suggests that stretching before certain intense exercises (basketball, tennis, soccer) can reduce muscle strain.

According to experts, what's key in the injury-prevention debate is how often you stretch. Habitual stretching that you do over a period of time, such as a yoga or stretch class, can reduce your risk of injury. But acute bouts of stretching, or stretching that you do only before and after your workouts, may not be as effective.

> Play It Safe

Keep these safety tips in mind when you stretch:

> Start slowly. It will become easier to stretch with practice.
> Don't force it. Overstretching can cause pain and injury. You might feel slight tension as you ease into a stretch, but it shouldn't hurt. If it does, stop.
> Breathe deeply. Don't hold your breath. Breathing slowly and deeply will help you relax and make stretching easier.
> Warm up. If you stretch before exercising, warm up your body for at least five

minutes first, with light movement such as walking or marching in place. You should avoid stretching a cold muscle, as you can increase your risk of pulling it.

> Stretch all major muscle groups, holding each stretch for at least 30 seconds. Fitness professionals recommend focusing on calf muscles, front and back thigh muscles (quadriceps and hamstrings), hip flexors, chest (pectoral) muscles and upper back muscles. You also can stretch your neck, shoulders, wrists and ankles.
> Stretch at least three times a week, if possible, and on most days that you exercise.
> Be careful about stretching after an injury; if you have a chronic illness, consult a doctor.
> Listen to your body and do what you can. Everyone has a different level of flexibility, which is partly determined by your genes.

> Stretching and More Stretching

Here are some activities you can try to improve your flexibility. They also can build strength, balance or both: yoga, pilates, ballet, modern dance, tai chi, martial arts, swimming and balance or stability ball.

If you're taking a class, give your body a chance to rest and repair itself by taking a day off from stretching. If you stretch as part of an exercise routine like walking or jogging, vary your stretches.

Stretching throughout the day, rather than in one longer time period, is perfectly okay, too. A couple of stretches in the morning after you get out of bed, in the evening when you get home from work, or at your desk at lunch or break time can re-energize mind and body. The more in tune you are with your body, the more active you want to be, experts say.

Whether you're trying to get active or have been active a long time, stretching will make you feel great all over. ■

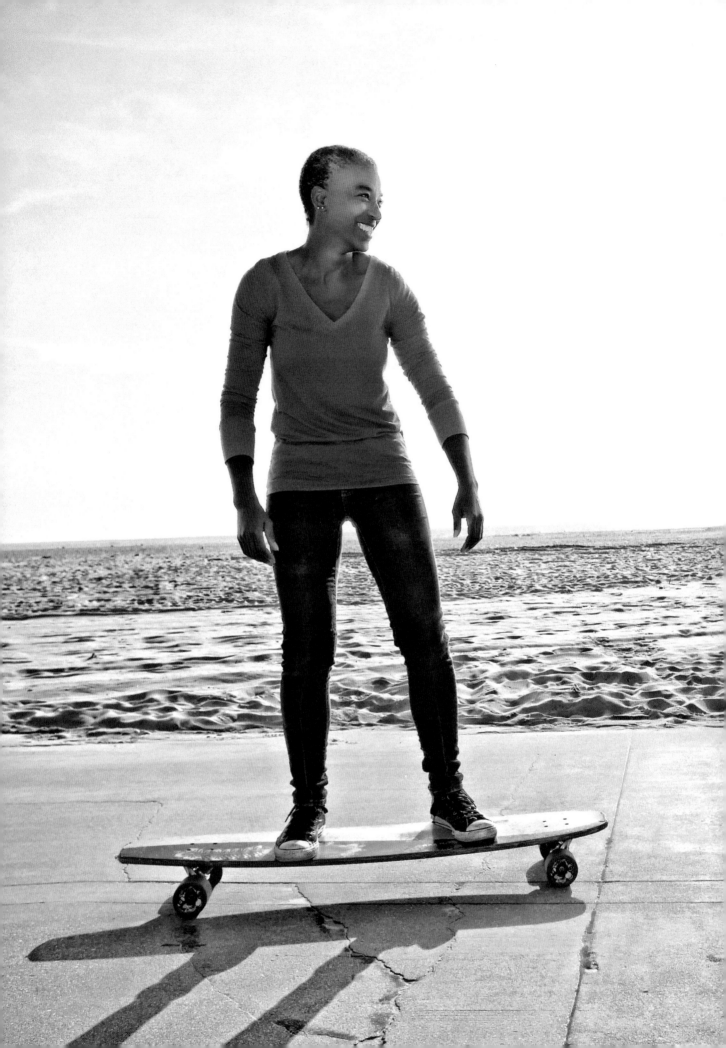

BONES AND JOINTS

EVERYTHING NEEDS A STRONG foundation and framework, and the body is no exception. Strong bones protect your organs and keep you mobile. Weak bones are more prone to fractures and breaks, which heal more slowly as we grow older. Bone and joint disease are associated with the later years of life, as are joint replacements, but none of these conditions is inevitable.

Bone is living tissue, and osteoporosis occurs when old bone breaks down faster than new bone is created. Osteoporosis affects an estimated 11 million Americans, and another 43 million have low bone mass. Osteoporosis causes bones to become so weak and brittle that even minor stresses can lead to breakage.

Arthritis, meanwhile, is a catch-all term for various types of joint pain and disease. More than 50 million Americans suffer from arthritis symptoms, including swelling, pain, stiffness and decreased range of motion. Severe arthritis can cause chronic pain, inability to perform particular tasks or enjoy activities, and permanent joint damage.

Calcium and vitamin D protect bones, but many of us don't get enough. This section explains why you need it, and how to get more of it in your diet (as well as what you should avoid). This section goes beyond a mere overview to also suggest nine dishes that will help you eat your way to stronger bones. We also provide information on how you can get—and keep—moving (with additional exercise tips in the Strength and Flexibility section), and when you should get tested and seek out medication.

The most important thing to remember when considering your bones? It is never too late to take care of your skeleton.

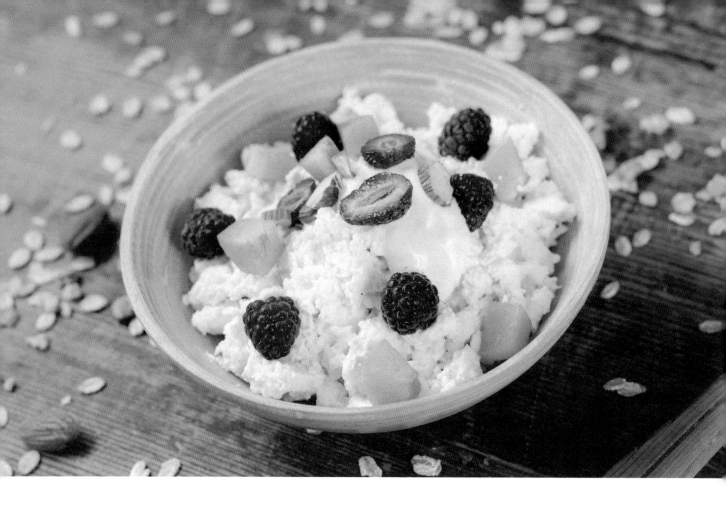

BOOST YOUR BONES AT ANY AGE

Diet, exercise and smart planning can give you the edge over osteoporosis

BY AMY PATUREL

STRONG BONES DON'T JUST protect against fractures from falls. They also improve your posture, protect your internal organs and give you the strength to do the things you love, from traveling to tai chi. Strong bones are also less prone to osteoporosis, which occurs when the body loses too much bone, makes too little bone, or both. About 54 million Americans have osteoporosis and low bone mass, and one in two women and up to one in four men age 50 and older will break a bone due to osteoporosis. While most of us reach peak bone mass by age 30, it's never too late to strengthen your structure. Here's how.

> **Get Milk**

Calcium and vitamin D help protect bones, but many Americans fall short on both nutrients. "If you're getting two to three servings of low-fat dairy every day and eating plenty of leafy greens, you should meet your calcium needs—1,000 milligrams for men and 1,200 for women," says Christine Gerbstadt, M.D., author of the *Doctor's Detox Diet*. Vitamin D is more difficult to obtain from food alone, though, even if you have a stellar diet. To get the recommended 600 to 800 international units daily, look for supplements that contain vitamin D3, an active form that's more effective than its vitamin D2 counterpart.

Quick tip: Lose the sugary soda. A study from Tufts University found that women who drink soda daily have lower bone mineral density than those who indulge only once a week. Scientists think the phosphoric acid in soda prevents calcium from being efficiently absorbed by your bones.

> Get Moving

Bones respond to stress by becoming denser and stronger. "The more impact on your bones, the better," says E. Michael Lewiecki, M.D., director of the New Mexico Clinical Research & Osteoporosis Center. Studies consistently show that athletes have up to 35 percent greater bone mineral content than nonathletes. Even simple activities such as walking and climbing stairs strengthen bones and muscles, improve balance and reduce your risk of falls. "Aim for at least 30 minutes of weight-bearing activity five to seven days a week to support your bones," suggests Heather Hofflich, associate clinical professor of medicine at UC San Diego Health.

Quick tip: Can't squeeze in a 30-minute workout? Incorporate push-ups and other strength-training activities into your day. You can even do lunges while you're doing other simple activites, like emptying the dishwasher, folding laundry or brushing your teeth.

> Get Tested

Men and women lose bone mass after age 50, but it's particularly noticeable when a woman enters menopause and bone-protecting hormones such as estrogen and progesterone plummet. "Women can lose as much as 5 to 10 percent of their bone mass in the first several years following menopause," says Lewiecki. If you fracture a bone, ask your doctor for a bone density test (a dual-energy X-ray absorptiometry, or DEXA, scan).

Quick tip: If you have thinning bones or are diagnosed with osteoporosis, bone-preserving medication, including bisphosphonates, which may help counteract some of the damage. ∎

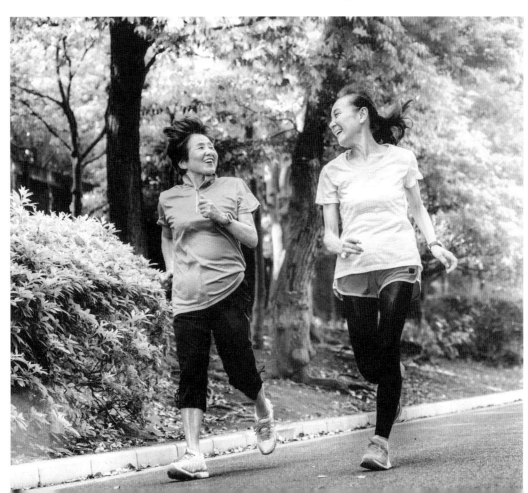

EAT YOUR WAY TO HEALTHY BONES

Explore calcium-rich meals

....

If you want to keep your bones strong and healthy, be sure to pay attention to what you eat. Although bone density begins to decline after age 50, if you maintain good nutrition, you may be far less vulnerable to bone thinning, fractures and breaks. The two crucial nutrients are calcium and vitamin D. You will find calcium in dairy products, of course, and also in dark green vegetables such as broccoli, cabbage, collard greens and kale (all of which provide a host of additional health benefits). Legumes are also good sources: foods with high calcium content include white beans, soybeans and Northern beans. Vitamin D, which helps your body absorb calcium, is found in eggs, liver, fortified dairy products, cereals and oily fish like salmon and sardines.

Preparing simple, healthy dishes like the ones presented here will help ensure you get the nutrients you need. If you don't have a favorite recipe on hand, research online until you find one that looks tempting. And keep these choices in mind when you're enjoying a night out at a restaurant, too. (Moderate exposure to sunlight is a calorie-free way to boost your vitamin D, so dine al fresco occasionally, or nab an outdoor table.) Don't forget that a bone-friendly lifestyle includes getting exercise, avoiding smoking and alcohol, and eating an overall healthy diet.

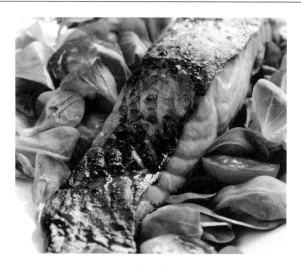

ROASTED SALMON

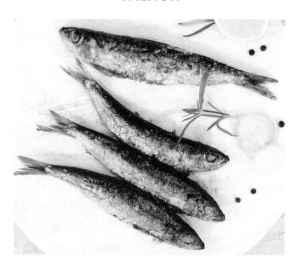

GRILLED SARDINES

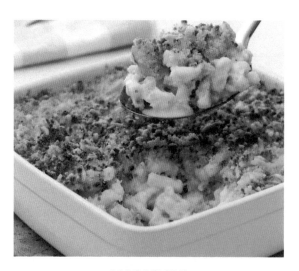

MACARONI AND CHEESE

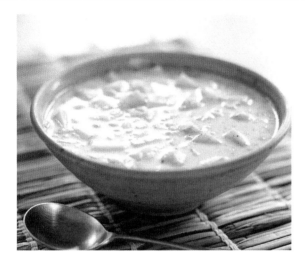

**CORN CHOWDER
WITH TROUT**

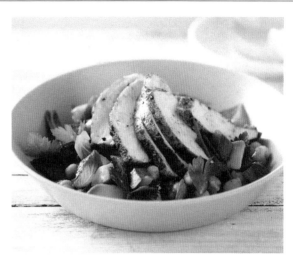

**CHICKEN BREASTS
WITH TOMATOES AND GARLIC**

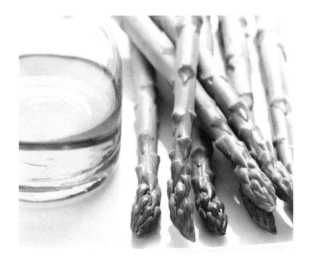

**ASPARAGUS WITH
GRATED CHEESE**

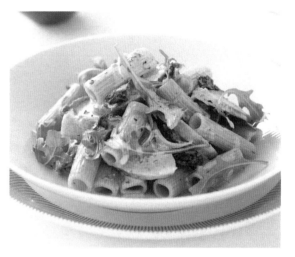

**PASTA WITH ARUGULA AND
SUN-DRIED TOMATOES**

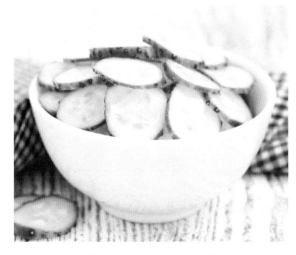

**CUCUMBER SALAD
WITH YOGURT DRESSING**

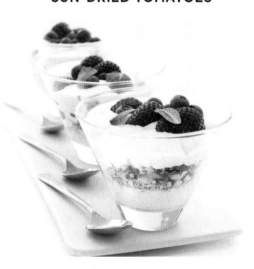

**YOGURT PARFAIT
WITH BERRIES**

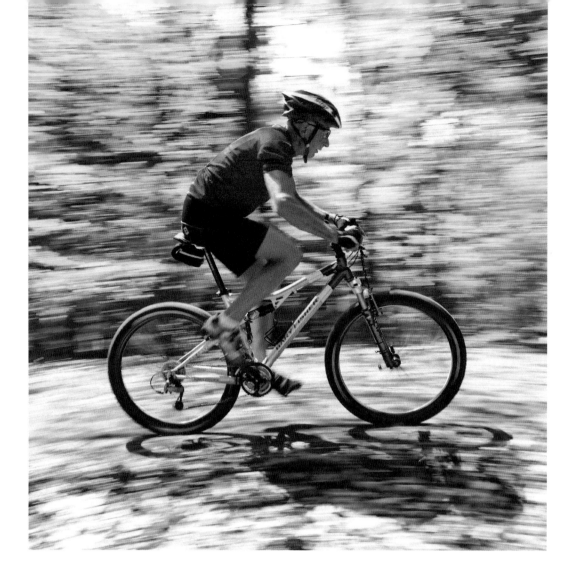

8 WAYS TO PREVENT ARTHRITIS

Here's what recent research suggests you should do

BY MEGHAN BOGARDUS

MILLIONS OF ADULTS OVER 50 live with arthritis—painful inflammation and stiffness of the joints. The parts of the body that are most often affected include the hand, spine, hip and knee. If you have arthritis, these suggestions could help you stay active and comfortable. If you don't have arthritis but you are at risk for or concerned about developing it, these tips are preventive, too.

> Get Moving

Maintaining a healthy weight and exercising regularly can help prevent some types of arthritis and lessen arthritis pain. Exercise strengthens muscles and joints, maintains flexibility and decreases fall risk. The most effective exercise regimen is a combination of aerobic exercise—think walking, biking and rowing—and strength training. Talk to your doctor before you start.

> Put a Cherry (or 10) on Top

Eating cherries, which contain powerful antioxidants with pain-fighting properties called anthocyanins, can lower the risk of gout, a type of arthritis. Study participants who ate at least 10 to 12 cherries over a two-day period had a 35 percent lower risk of flare-ups, the journal *Arthritis & Rheumatism* reports. Research also suggests that drinking tart cherry juice may ease some osteoarthritis pain.

A compound found in extra virgin olive oil may work like ibuprofen to ease arthritis pain.

> Skip Sodas

Sugary soft drinks not only add to weight gain but may also contribute to the progression of knee osteoarthritis, especially in men who drink more than five sodas a week, according to research at Brigham and Women's Hospital and Tufts Medical Center. Sodas also may up the risk of rheumatoid arthritis in women, Harvard researchers concluded in a 2014 study.

> Pass on Prime Rib

Eating foods high in purines—especially organ meats like liver, but also other meat and animal products as well as oily fish and shellfish, spinach and mushrooms—can make gout flare-ups almost five times more likely than if you eat low-purine foods, finds an *Annals of the Rheumatic Diseases* study.

> Go Alternative

Acupuncture and tai chi have been shown to be effective treatments for pain caused by rheumatoid arthritis, according to a study at the University of Aberdeen in Scotland. Massage may also offer some relief from joint pain. Be sure to talk to your doctor before beginning complementary medicine treatment.

> Choose Olive Oil

A growing body of research suggests that a compound found in extra virgin olive oil may reduce inflammation caused by rheumatoid arthritis. In fact, it appears to work much like ibuprofen to ease arthritis pain. So, use it in a salad dressing, toss it with spaghetti, or drip on vegetables. Just go easy—it's healthy, but it's also heavy on calories.

> Enjoy a Cocktail

Women who consumed more than three alcoholic drinks a week over a 10-year period reduced their risk of rheumatoid arthritis by about half, according to a study in the *British Medical Journal*. But choose your drink wisely. Beer may increase your risk of knee and hip osteoarthritis. No matter what you drink, avoid overindulging. Excess alcohol also ups your risk of developing gout. ∎

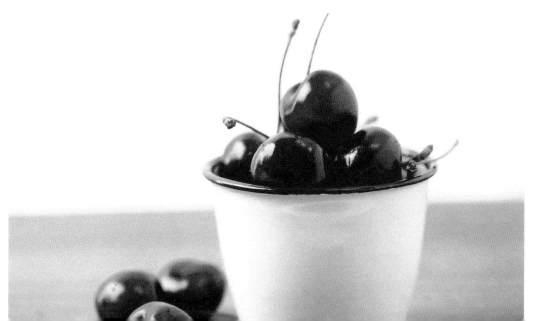

MIND

MANY OF US THINK OF THE mind and body as separate entities, even though the brain is housed in our physical form. The truth is, the mind and body are inextricably intertwined in countless ways. If the brain is not sharp, the rest of the body suffers. If the other organs and the bones and muscles are not functioning well, the mind will be affected. To experience our happiest, fullest lives, we must take care to keep our minds operating at peak levels.

The most common symptom associated with the brain is loss of memory, and it's an issue that worries many of us. As ever, eating a healthy diet and keeping physically and mentally active can help keep memory issues at bay. This section begins by examining six types of memory lapses that are not cause for alarm, from hunting for your keys to getting details confused to struggling to recall a new friend's name. Next, we move on to exploring the benefits of playing simple games. No need to purchase an expensive computer program or force-feed yourself crossword puzzles; playing Concentration or another basic card game can stimulate the brain and even boost the immune system.

Finally, we walk you through how to improve your brain health in just one day, with suggestions every hour to sharpen your complex reasoning skills, boost your memory, and enhance concentration. You can start with a brisk walk upon waking up, rearrange your surroundings midmorning, and doodle after a lunch of healthy greens. In the evening, focus on mindfulness and settle on your side to help your brain clear out toxins that have accumulated during the day. You don't need to study neuroscience to keep your brain sharp; a little effort will keep your noggin humming—and help you maintain your overall health as well.

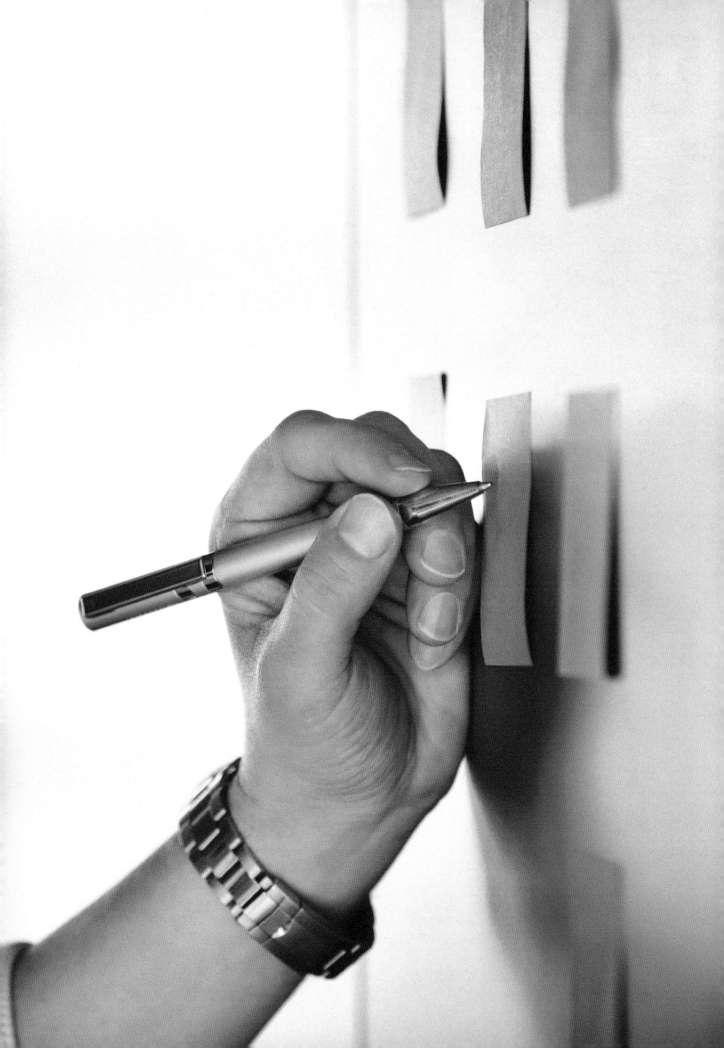

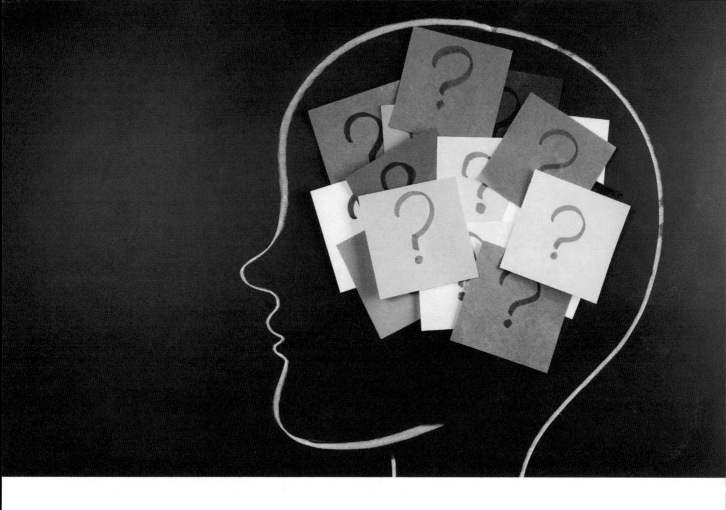

NORMAL MEMORY PROBLEMS

Common issues—and why you needn't worry about them

BY MARY A. FISCHER

MAYBE IT STARTS WITH SIMPLY forgetting something, like you can't remember the route to a restaurant you've been to many times before or the birthday present a friend gave you a month ago. Then comes the worry. Is your forgetfulness a sign of something serious? Such brain freezes happen to most of us, to different degrees, as we age. Even experienced public speakers have their "oops" moments, when a word or term they use on a daily basis simply refuses to come to mind.

But while such common memory lapses are frustrating, they don't necessarily mean you're losing your marbles. If your lapses aren't dis-rupting your life, there's no need to be actively worried, experts say. "The key issue is whether cognitive changes are significantly interfering with daily activities," says Kirk R. Daffner, M.D., chief of the division of cognitive and behavioral neurology at Boston's Brigham and Women's Hospital. If that's happening, you should consult your doctor. Your lapses may well have very treat-able causes. Severe stress, depression, a vitamin B-12 deficiency, insufficient sleep, some prescrip-tion drugs and infections can all play a role.

Even if these factors don't apply to you, your memory isn't completely at the mercy of time. Studies have shown that people who exercise,

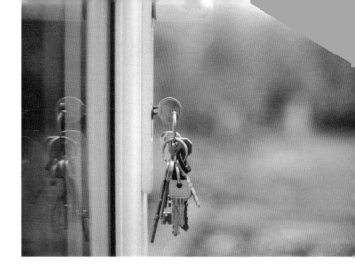

stay mentally active, socialize regularly and eat a healthy diet can minimize memory loss. Still worried? Here are six types of normal memory lapses that are not a cause for worry.

1 Absentmindedness.

Where in the world did you leave your keys? Or why the heck did you walk into the living room anyway? Both of these very common lapses usually stem from lack of attention or focus. It's perfectly normal to forget directions to somewhere you haven't visited in a while. But "if you've lived on a block for 10 years, and you walk out the door and get lost, that's much more serious," says Debra Babcock, M.D., of the National Institute of Neurological Disorders and Stroke.

2 Blocking.

This is the frustrating tip-of-the-tongue moment. You know the word you're trying to say, but you can't quite retrieve it from memory. It usually happens when several similar memories interfere with each other. A recent study, published in the journal *Brain Research*, showed that elderly participants had to activate more areas of the brain to perform a memory task than the study's young subjects. "We're all accessing the same brain networks to remember things," says Babcock, "but we have to call in the troops to do the work when we get older, while we only have to call in a few soldiers when we're younger."

3 Misattribution.

This is when you accurately remember most of an event or other chunk of information, but confuse certain key details. One example: A good friend tells you over dinner at a restaurant that she is taking out a second mortgage on her home. Later, you correctly recall the gist of her news but think she told you during a phone conversation. Research points to the importance of the hippocampus—a region of the brain crucial in the formation of memories about events, including the particular time and place they occurred. Scientists estimate that, after the age of about 25, the hippocampus loses 5 percent of its nerve cells with each passing decade.

4 Fading away.

The brain is always sweeping out older memories to make room for new ones. The more time that passes between an experience and when you want to recall it, the more likely you are to have forgotten much of it. So while it is typically fairly easy to remember what you did over the past several hours, recalling the same events and activities a month, or a year, later is considerably more difficult. This basic "use-it-or-lose-it" feature of memory known as transience is normal at all ages, not just among older adults.

5 Struggling for retrieval.

You were just introduced to someone, and seconds later, you can't remember her name. Or you saw a great film, but when you tell a friend about it the next day, you've completely forgotten the title. Aging changes the strengths of the connections between neurons in the brain. New information can bump out other items from short-term memory unless it is repeated again and again.

6 Muddled multitasking.

Multitasking isn't as productive as we may think, no matter your age. So maybe you can't watch the news and talk on the phone at the same time anymore. Not such a bad thing, really. Studies show that, the older we get, the more the brain has to exert effort to maintain focus. Further, it takes longer to get back to an original task after an interruption. ■

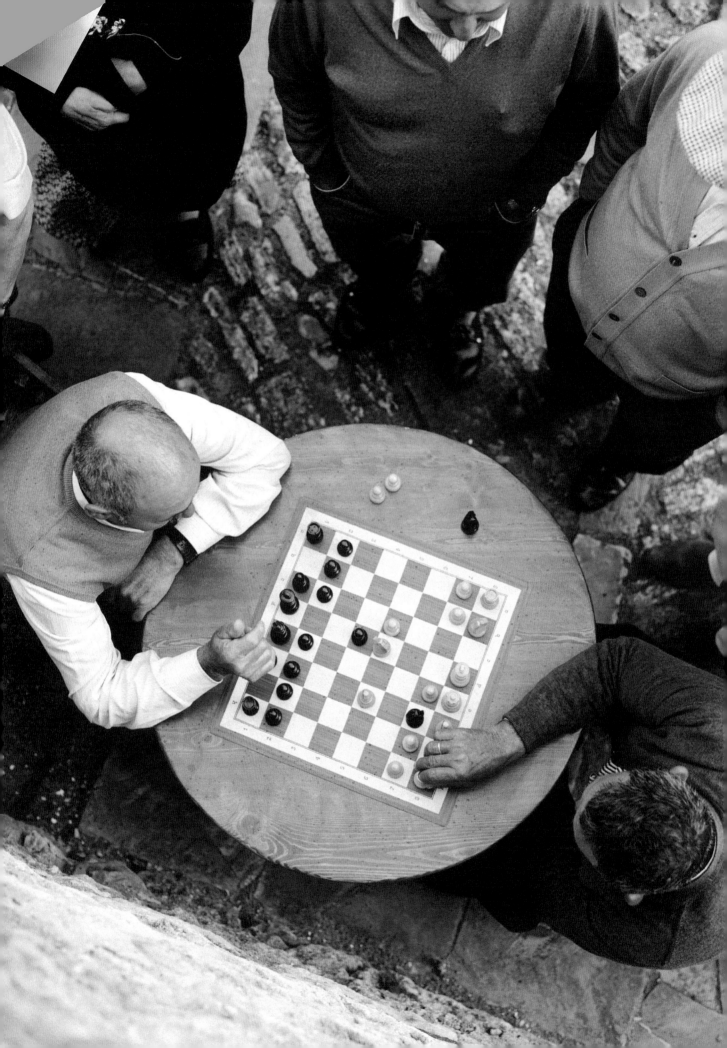

CAN CHESS HELP YOUR BRAIN?

Mental stimulation may help with problem-solving and lower the risk of Alzheimer's

BY RENÉE BACHER

PLAYING GAMES MAY BE GOOD for brain health, and it can be the inexpensive, old-fashioned kind of games, not just those requiring a computer and a subscription to activities created by neuroscientists. Multiple studies have shown associations between different forms of cognitive mental stimulation and better brain health, whether it's playing cards, reading books, engaging in stimulating conversations or learning. And all of these seem to be associated with a lower risk for Alzheimer's disease.

Working memory, which we use to recall things we need for only seconds or minutes (such as what everyone wants on their pizza before we place the order), is important for many tasks, including those requiring creativity and problem solving. Although our working memory tends to wane as we age, we can boost it with frequent use, and that has more than just short-term value. "It turns out this has a transfer effect to improving what's called fluid intelligence, a form of IQ we use when problem solving," says Gary Small, M.D., director of the UCLA Longevity Center, coauthor of *2 Weeks to a Younger Brain* and author of *The Mind Health Report* monthly newsletter. Fluid intelligence is an aspect of IQ we use when problem solving. "You've got to hold bits of information in your mind to navigate to the solution," Small says.

Even the simplest games, such as Concentration, designed for children, can strengthen working memory. Each card has a matching image, all cards are placed face down and players take turns turning over two cards at each turn in the hopes of discovering a pair. One study suggested that playing bridge (which requires opponents to use higher-order functions, such as planning ahead, sorting and sequencing cards) stimulates the dorsolateral cortex—responsible for working memory, cognitive flexibility, decision making and other executive functions—as well as the thymus gland, which produces T cells that assist the immune system in finding viruses, among other things that can make us sick. Take the time to have a little fun—and do some good for your brain, as well. ■

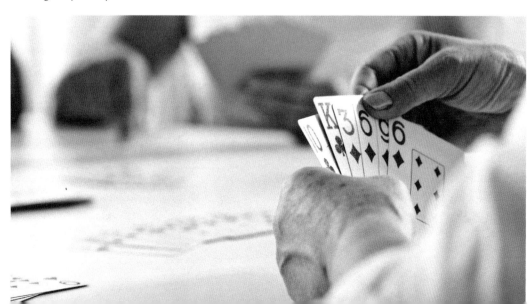

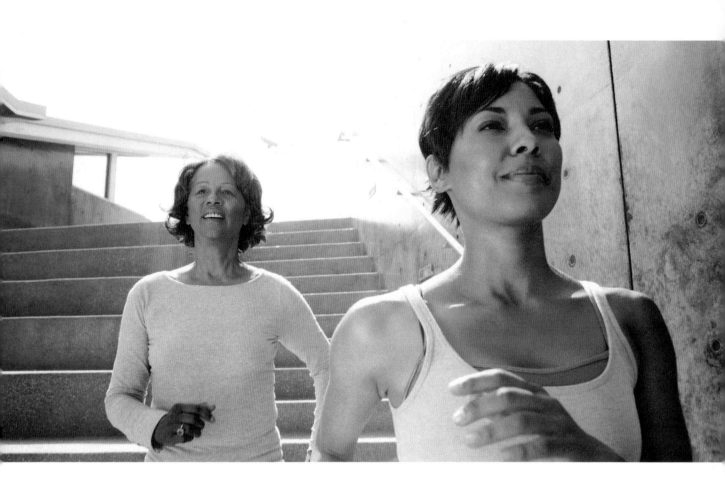

BOOST YOUR BRAIN IN 24 HOURS

An hour-by-hour guide to feeding, challenging and enhancing your brain

BY ROBIN WESTEN

THINK YOUR BEST DAYS OF CRE-ativity, innovation and productivity are behind you? Not so. Exciting new research finds that our complex reasoning skills can sharpen as we age, provided we give our brains the proper nourishment and stimulation.

"The latest research shows that if you challenge your brain every day with novel activities, support its health with important nutrients, and regularly exercise to bring it oxygen and blood, your intellect can improve, no matter what your age," says Glenn Smith, Ph.D., chair of the department of clinical and health psychology at the University of Florida and emeritus professor of psychology at the Mayo Clinic College of Medicine in Rochester,

Minnesota. Try these simple suggestions to help boost your memory and enhance your concentration throughout the day.

⊕ 6 a.m. Get up and get moving

A brisk walk (not a leisurely stroll) three times a week can increase the size of your hippocampus—the brain's command center for memories. "Walking pumps oxygen and nutrients to your brain cells and builds brain 'muscles,'" says Gary Small, M.D., director of the UCLA Longevity Center, and author to coauthor of *2 Weeks to a Younger Brain*. Get even more mental perks by walking in a park or down a country road; spending time in nature elevates mood and memory.

🕐 **7 a.m.** Chill out That warm bath might feel good, but a cool shower might be better for your brain. Researchers at the Virginia Commonwealth University School of Medicine found that a chilly shower stimulates the "blue spot," the brain's primary source of noradrenaline, a chemical that helps alleviate the blues. That's important because of the well-known links between depression and cognitive decline.

🕐 **8 a.m.** Grab some java People who drink one to two cups of caffeinated coffee a day have a lower rate of mild cognitive impairment than do those who never or rarely drink the stuff, according to a 2015 study in the *Journal of Alzheimer's Disease*. Give your brain an extra edge by pairing that cup of joe with some yogurt. University of California, Los Angeles, researchers concluded that women who regularly eat probiotics (look for yogurt with "live and active cultures") have improved brain function both while resting and when completing tasks to recognize various emotions.

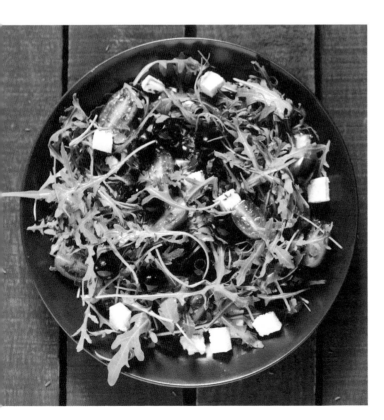

🕐 **9 a.m.** Pencil it in Are you a gadget kind of guy or gal? New research in *Psychological Science* finds that taking notes with pencil (or pen) and paper—rather than always using a computer—strengthens your memory and your ability to understand challenging concepts. Keep a pad of paper or a notebook handy to give your brain a mini workout.

🕐 **10 a.m.** Rearrange the furniture Your brain gets bored when faced with the same environment every day. Knock it out of its comfort zone by moving things around—literally. You don't need to redesign the whole house—move a few pictures, or just turn your desk photos upside down. This kind of mental exercise, dubbed neurobics, challenges your brain by forcing it to make new neural connections, says Ron Frostig, professor of neurobiology and behavior at the University of California, Irvine.

🕐 **11 a.m.** Stop multitasking You already know that multitasking decreases your productivity—by as much as 40 percent, researchers say. Scarier still, this can temporarily lower your IQ in the bargain, scientists at the University of London have discovered. Participants in a study who multitasked while trying to solve cognitive problems scored nearly 10 points lower, on average, on an IQ test. Instead of juggling, tackle your tasks one at a time. You'll be more productive and more relaxed.

🕐 **12 p.m.** Go green A daily salad featuring dark leafy greens such as spinach, kale, collards, Swiss chard and mustard greens offers serious brain benefits, note researchers at Rush University Medical Center in Chicago. The scientists followed the eating habits and cognitive function of more than 950 older adults for five years and found that those who had one to two servings a day of leafy greens had the cognitive function of people 11 years younger. Brain-healthy add-ons—including salmon, olive oil and walnuts—could boost your brain health even more.

🕐 **1 p.m.** Hit save Can a computer's storage help extend your own memory bank? It sounds futuristic, but research from the University of California, Santa Cruz, indicates it's happening now. All you may need to do to improve your memory is to regularly hit Save on the computer. Study participants were given seconds to study a PDF with nouns listed on it. After that time elapsed, they were told to close the file and begin studying a second, similar file. Half of the people were also told to save the first PDF to a specific folder on their computer before moving on to the second task. This group was consistently able to recall more words from the second file than were those who didn't press Save on the first. The scientists concluded that when data is saved on a computer, your brain learns to off-load it from active memory. In essence, this gives the brain a break so it can process new information more efficiently.

🕐 **2 p.m.** Peek at a screen saver Looking at an image of a scenic view can improve your concentration. And you don't have to do it for long. In a recent study, researchers from the University of Melbourne in Australia found that interrupting a tedious, demanding chore with a mere 40-second gaze at an image of a flowering-meadow green roof substantially improved the participants' focus when they returned to their task.

🕐 **3 p.m.** Scribble during meetings Doodles aren't only for distracted daydreamers. Those squiggles can help you remember information. Researchers at the University of Plymouth in England asked study participants to listen to a message about an upcoming party and then write down the names of folks who were going to attend—and those who were not. Half the participants were additionally given instructions to doodle while writing down the names; the other half were told to write down the names only, no doodling. The result? Doodlers later recalled 30 percent more names and places.

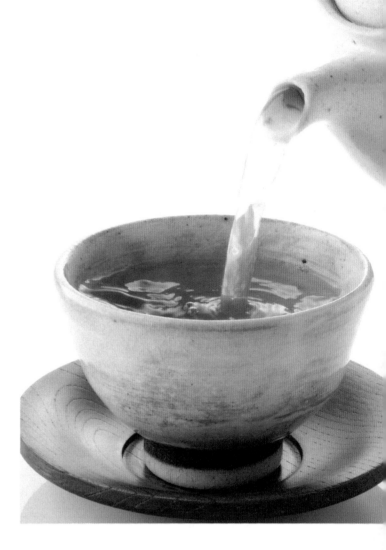

🕐 **4 p.m.** Take 10 for tea Sipping green tea instead of black can benefit your brain big-time. A study presented at the 12th International Conference on Alzheimer's and Parkinson's Diseases showed that people who drink green tea one to six days a week have less mental decline than those who don't. Some researchers speculate that this may be due to L-theanine, an amino acid found in green tea, which increases levels of the brain chemicals gamma-aminobutyric acid (GABA), serotonin and dopamine, plus bumps up alpha wave activity, all of which may help to prevent age-related memory decline and enhance areas of the brain involved in complex thinking and concentration.

🕐 **5 p.m.** Flex your noodle Don't be put off by the directions that follow. Once you get the hang of this yoga brain exercise, it takes just three minutes (tops) to complete. The exercise—based on research at the Department of Radiological Sciences at the University of California—involves using the body's major acupuncture points to synchronize the right and left hemispheres of the brain, which can encourage faster thought processing. Give it a try.

> Remove any jewelry.
> Face north.
> Rest your tongue against the roof of your mouth throughout the exercise.
> With your left hand, grasp your right earlobe with thumb and forefinger. Make sure your thumb is in front.
> With your right hand, grasp your left earlobe; again, be sure your thumb is in front. At this point, you're pressing both earlobes simultaneously.
> Inhale through your nose and slowly squat.
> Hold your breath and exhale as you start returning to a standing position.
> Repeat this squatting action 14 times. Remember to hold your earlobes and keep your tongue against the roof of your mouth throughout the exercise.

⊕ **6 p.m.** Make it Italian tonight Older adults who followed a Mediterranean-style diet—with an emphasis on whole grains, vegetables, fruit, fish, beans, cereals and the occasional serving of chicken—had more gray matter, a study in *Neurology* concluded. The bigger brain volume equaled about five years of brain aging, researchers say.

⊕ **7 p.m.** Get your mindfulness on Mindfulness-based stress reduction can significantly improve quality of life for people with mild cognitive impairment (MCI), according to findings from Beth Israel Deaconess Medical Center in Boston. A group of adults with MCI, ages 55 to 90, did a guided mindful meditation and movement for 30 minutes a day for eight weeks, and attended weekly mindfulness check-ins. Eight

weeks later, they showed an overall improvement in cognition and well-being. A simple meditation technique involves sitting in a chair with your posture as straight as possible, closing your eyes and counting your breaths. If thoughts come in—and they will—don't try to stop them. Instead, imagine they're passing clouds; let them go and return to your breath.

⊕ **8 p.m.** Say no to nibbling If you make a habit of late-night grazing, your weight isn't the only thing that will suffer—your brain might, too. A UCLA study looked at the eating habits of mice and found that the equivalent of snacking into the wee hours impaired their ability to learn new information as well as to store memories. What's the connection? The researchers concluded that the rodents' irregular eating schedule interfered with the rhythm of the hippocampus, which regulates memories.

⊕ **9 p.m.** Let it go Are you worried you're becoming forgetful? It's time to stop ruminating about it. "A perfect day for brain health also includes avoiding depression, anger and anxiety," says David Knopman M.D., a Mayo Clinic neurologist. The anxiety you're feeling, it turns out, will only make your memory worse, a North Carolina State University study published in *Psychology and Aging* found. Participants who were told that aging causes forgetfulness scored poorly on memory tests, whereas those who were told there isn't much of a decline in later years did 30 percent better.

⊕ **10 p.m.** Become a side sleeper Sleeping on your side, as opposed to your stomach or back, allows the brain to clear toxic chemicals more efficiently, according to researchers at Stony Brook University in New York. That's important because chemicals and waste that build up in the brain have been associated with Alzheimer's and Parkinson's. Plus, research suggests that most people need six to eight hours of sleep nightly to effectively clear out brain toxins. ■

HEART

THE HEART IS, BY DEFINITION, the center of it all. Cardiovascular health is paramount throughout our entire lives, and it gets a lot of attention as we grow older. This section walks you through some new and interesting information: unexpected factors that may affect your ticker; foods that can improve your heart health; and high-tech devices and procedures that can give you a boost—or save your life.

It's old news that too much weight, too little exercise, high blood pressure, stress and smoking may lead to heart disease and even fatal heart attacks. But additional factors can take a toll on the body and cause cardiovascular issues. Common medications—like those for asthma, heartburn and everyday aches and pains—are associated with heart attack. In some cases, the medication itself can cause a problem; in others, the drugs are associated with systemic problems (like asthma) that may indicate increased risks for your heart. Similarly, if you suffer from particular headaches, set your clocks ahead in spring or fail to contain your anger, your heart may be more vulnerable. Learn what might indicate a problem, and what you can do to be more vigilant.

Foods with omega-3 fatty acids have enjoyed a good reputation for some time, but recent research has proven that they can significantly lower your chances of dying from a heart attack. We explain exactly what the latest news reveals, and lay out the best sources for adding more of these foods to your diet.

And if the best in preventive care is not enough to keep heart disease at bay, it's important to know the latest in new treatments and procedures. Exciting new innovations like heart regeneration, beating-heart transplants, minimally invasive valve replacement and a beatless heart can extend your life—and vastly improve the quality of your years.

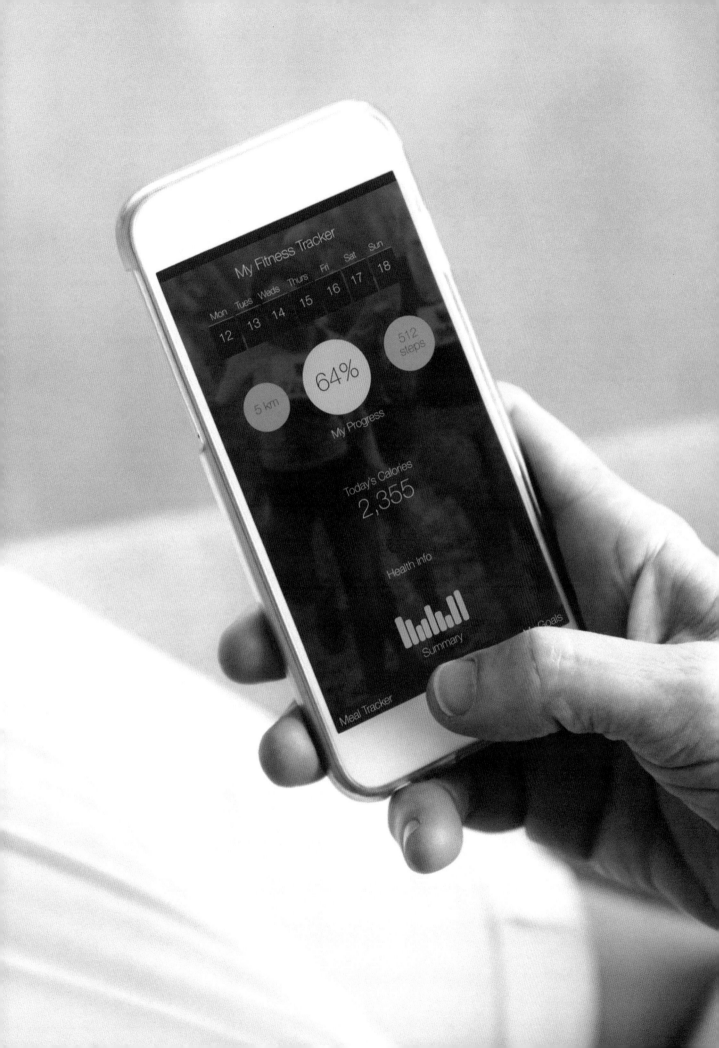

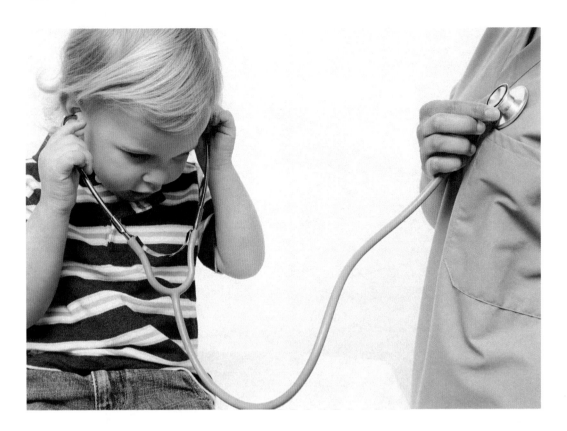

TIPS FOR A HEALTHIER HEART

Watch out for these unexpected potential cardio triggers

BY JODI HELMER

WHEN IT COMES TO HEART attacks, many of us know the causes most likely to trigger a problem: obesity, not enough exercise, high blood pressure, stress and smoking. But new research is finding other, less common factors may also put your heart at risk. Check with your doctor about the latest research.

1 Asthma requiring daily medication.
Asthma severe enough to require daily controller medications is associated with a 60 percent higher risk of a heart attack, stroke or death from cardiovascular disease, as both asthma and heart disease are associated with high levels of inflammation.

2 Taking certain heartburn drugs.
Taking proton pump inhibitors (PPIs) was associated with a 16 to 21 percent higher heart attack risk. PPIs may reduce the production of nitric oxide, an important molecule that helps maintain the health of the inner linings of blood vessels.

3 Having migraines with aura.
Middle-aged and older women who have migraines with aura (also known as classic

migranes) have an increased risk of heart attack. Migraine with aura was found to be the second-strongest contributor to heart attack and stroke risk after high blood pressure. These migraine sufferers should try to reduce their risk in other ways, including not smoking, staying active and keeping blood pressure under control.

4 Skipping the flu vaccine.

A flu vaccine also helps your heart, decreasing your odds of having a heart attack by 50 percent in the year following the shot compared with those who don't get the vaccine. Antibodies that are produced after the vaccination activate molecular processes, which protect and strengthen the cardiovascular system.

5 Weak grip strength.

Researchers found that grip strength is as strong (and may be better) a predictor of cardiac death as blood pressure. While the cause of the link is unknown, there could be a connection between muscle strength and improved vascular function.

6 Daylight Saving Time.

Research presented at the American College of Cardiology's 63rd Annual Scientific Session noted a 25 percent increase in the number of heart attacks on the Monday after the clocks move ahead—or "spring forward"—and we lose an hour, compared with other Mondays during the year. The sleep disruption from the spring time change is stressful to the body, and may trigger a heart attack in susceptible patients.

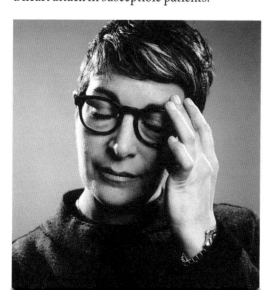

7 The cocktail hour.

When it comes to whether alcohol helps or hurts heart health, timing appears to be everything. For those who do not drink regularly, the chances of having a heart attack increased 72 percent in the first hour after drinking alcohol. Within the first hour after drinking, your heart rate and blood pressure increase, and your blood becomes more sticky, making it more likely to clot.

8 Anger issues.

If you're blowing your top at every little thing, those outbursts are sending your heart attack risk skyrocketing. Even if you can't prevent anger entirely, lowering how often you get angry or lowering the intensity can be helpful for lowering your heart attack risk.

9 Traumatic events.

Traumatic life events like the death of a loved one or a life-threatening illness increased heart attack risk by nearly 70 percent among middle-aged and older women. Negative experiences might interfere with the body's response to stress, increasing inflammation and stress hormones, which are linked to susceptibility to heart attacks.

10 Taking common painkillers.

The widely used painkillers ibuprofen and naproxen come with a warning that they "may cause" an increased risk of heart problems, but new data convinced the FDA to strengthen the wording to say these medications "cause" a higher risk, and the agency warns that Americans should use the drugs sparingly for a brief time, and at the lowest dose possible. New studies show the risk of heart attack or stroke can increase even after a short period of usage. The risk also appears greater at higher doses. People who have heart disease, particularly those who recently had a heart attack or cardiac bypass surgery, are at the greatest risk and should discuss taking these drugs with their doctor. ■

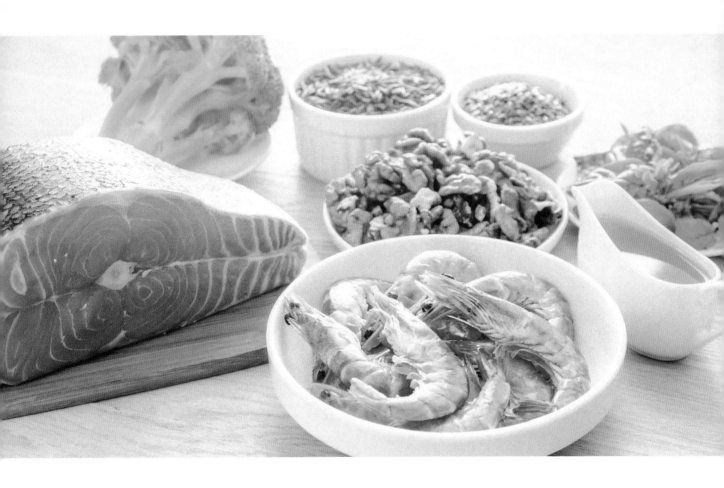

HEART-HAPPY FOODS WITH OMEGA-3 OILS

Here's what you need to eat to get the most benefits for your heart

BY CANDY SAGON

WHEN IT COMES TO OMEGA-3 fatty acids, like the kind found in fish oil, the big question has been whether they really help prevent heart disease. Findings up to now have been frustratingly mixed, but a new comprehensive analysis of international studies suggests a clearer answer: Regularly eating fish, nuts and other omega-3-rich foods is associated with a significantly lower risk of dying from a heart attack.

"Our results lend support to the importance of fish and omega-3 consumption as part of a healthy diet," says senior study author Dariush Mozaffarian, dean of the Friedman School of Nutrition Science and Policy at Tufts University.

The new research, published in the journal *JAMA Internal Medicine*, avoided some of the pitfalls of previous studies, many of which relied on self-reported food consumption or were conducted on people who already had heart disease.

Instead, a group of international researchers analyzed large studies that had measured blood or tissue levels of omega-3 fatty acids, avoiding the problems of bias or error involved in subjects recalling what they ate. The researchers also excluded study participants with any prior heart disease or stroke.

A total of 19 studies from 16 countries involving nearly 46,000 adults (ages 18 to 97) were analyzed. Overall, eating a diet rich in fish and plant foods (such as nuts and seeds)—but not taking fish oil pills, which few participants did—was associated with about a 10 percent lower risk of fatal heart attacks overall. People with the highest blood levels of omega-3s had about a 25 percent lower risk of fatal heart attack, compared to people with the lowest levels.

The findings were also consistent across age, sex, race, presence or absence of diabetes, and use of aspirin or statins, researchers reported, although the study can't prove a cause-and-effect. "These new results, which include many studies which previously had not reported their findings, provide the most comprehensive picture to-date of how omega-3s may influence heart disease," said co-author Liana Del Gobbo, a researcher with the Stanford Prevention Research Center in the Department of Medicine at Stanford University. ∎

GOOD SOURCES

To add more omega-3s to your diet, here are some of the top sources:

Fish The best choices are salmon (fresh or canned), tuna (fresh or canned), trout, halibut, canned sardines, mackerel (fresh or canned) and oysters.

Eggs Look for those from hens fed a diet fortified with omega-3 fatty acids (it will say so on the label). The eggs will have more omega-3s in the yolk.

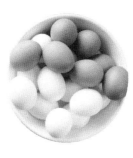

Nuts Many nuts contain omega-3s, including fortified peanut butter, but the champion is walnuts, which contain the most.

Grass-fed beef This contains about three times as much omega-3 fatty acids as corn-fed beef, but not nearly as much as fish.

Seeds Flax seeds are rich sources of omega-3 fats. Chia and hemp seeds are also good sources. Sunflower seeds have a small amount.

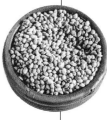

Some vegetables Cauliflower, Brussels sprouts, kale, broccoli, arugula, summer squash and collard greens can also contribute omega-3s to your diet.

Tofu and edamame Boiled, shelled green soybeans (edamame) and tofu are good sources of omega-3s.

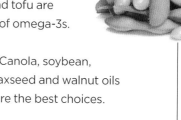

Oils Canola, soybean, flaxseed and walnut oils are the best choices.

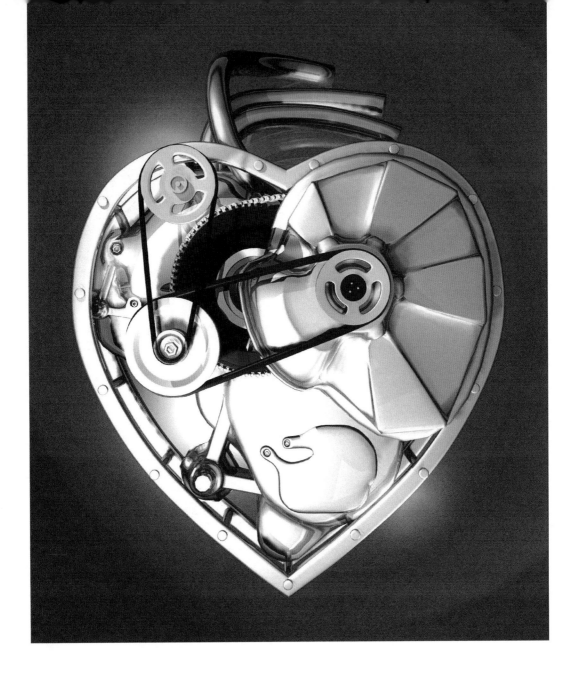

HIGH-TECH HEART SAVERS

These innovative new procedures could save your life

BY AMY PATUREL

WITH HEART DISEASE AF-fecting an estimated 28 million adults—nearly 12 percent of the U.S. population—researchers are racing to develop new treatments.

> Heart Regeneration

During most heart attacks, a blood clot forms and blocks one of the coronary arteries that feed the heart. This kills part of the heart muscle, turning it into scar tissue, which often leads to shortness of breath, weakness and a reduced ability to exercise. Today researchers at the Cedars-Sinai Heart Institute in Los Angeles are using a patient's bone marrow stem cells to transform scar tissue into living heart muscle. The idea is simple: Harvest stem cells from an unaffected part of the heart, multiply them in the laboratory and inject them into the site of the injury, so they can take root and repair the damage.

Heart attack survivors treated with their own stem cells within three months of an attack experienced a 50 percent reduction in scar tissue, on average, and all generated new heart tissue. Multiple advanced stem cell trials are ongoing, and results are impressive and promising.

> Beating-Heart Transplants

When a donor heart is ready for transplant, it's typically packed in a picnic cooler with a bag of cold saline solution. Cheap and easy, maybe, but also inefficient, since donor hearts begin to deteriorate the moment they're removed from a person's chest.

Bruce Rosengard, M.D., chief technology officer for global surgery at Johnson & Johnson, pushed to make the beating-heart transplant a reality. Here's how it works: A miniature machine circulates donor blood through the heart until moments before it's stitched into a recipient's chest.

Recovery time is promising, too. In a European study, 19 of 20 patients who received beating-heart transplants were out of the intensive care unit in less than 24 hours; the twentieth patient was out in under 48 hours. Standard transplants, by comparison, typically require at least two days in the ICU.

> Minimally Invasive Valve Replacement

Heart valves, like joints, break down over time because of wear and tear. And every year about 50,000 patients undergo complex open-heart surgery to receive new ones. Now doctors have developed a procedure to replace ailing valves without cutting open a patient's chest.

The procedure, called transcatheter aortic valve replacement, or TAVR, uses a catheter to guide the artificial valve to the beating heart through a small incision in the leg or between the ribs. "It's far less traumatic than open-heart surgery, especially for patients who are inoperable or high risk," says Alan C. Yeung, M.D., chief of the division of cardiovascular medicine at Stanford. In fact, surgeons can't perform the procedure if the person's heart is young and healthy. "We rely on defects in the heart—spots that are hardened—to hold the valve in place," he explains. The new valve expands and pushes the old valve aside.

The FDA approved the breakthrough procedure in 2011, after a two-year follow-up study showed it reduced the risk of death by more than 40 percent. A bonus: TAVR can take as little as an hour, and patients are awake and talking within a couple of hours.

> A Beatless Heart

Each year up to 40,000 patients would benefit from a heart transplant, yet only about 2,200 donor hearts are available. Artificial hearts are a time-tested alternative (they've been available since 1982), but the primary model, the Jarvik-7, requires the use of an external air compressor, and patients need maintenance surgeries, which carry risks and take a toll on the body.

A team at the Texas Heart Institute in Houston has introduced a new device, called a beatless heart, that pushes blood through the body at a steady rate, like a Jet Ski propeller. With no valves, flexible components or complex machinery, it acts less like a heart than a pair of turbines, says inventor William Cohn, M.D., director of minimally invasive surgical technology at the institute. It doesn't burn out as fast as an artificial heart with multiple parts.

Plans are under way to test the device (and procedure) in a half-dozen human patients. If the technology shows promise, Cohn's team hopes to begin clinical trials soon after, though it predicts that FDA approval is several years away. ∎

SLEEP

SLEEP IS, IN MANY WAYS, THE cornerstone of a healthy body. No matter how well we eat, how frequently we exercise and how well we attend to every aspect of our health, it is all for naught if we are not well rested.

Chronic sleep deprivation takes a toll on our physical, mental and even spiritual health; it affects every system in the body. Poor sleep leads to immediate negative effects as well as chronic issues over the long term. As we grow older, our sleep patterns change. We may go to sleep and rise much earlier than when we were young, and we may have more trouble falling and staying asleep. Older people also tend to spend more time in lighter sleep phases and less time in deep sleep.

This section explores the importance of sleep, then focuses on concrete steps you can take right now to improve the quality of your sleep. The right foods and exercise are essential, of course, but it's also important to establish a routine, get outdoors and consider when you take your medications.

If your circadian rhythms are off, we can help you reset your internal clock to get back on track. Some tips include considering what you put in your mouth and when; being mindful of when your body needs light and when it requires darkness; fitting your activities around your body's natural schedule; and using your computer to jump-start your brain. Even if you've long since despaired of getting a good night's sleep, rest easy: We can help.

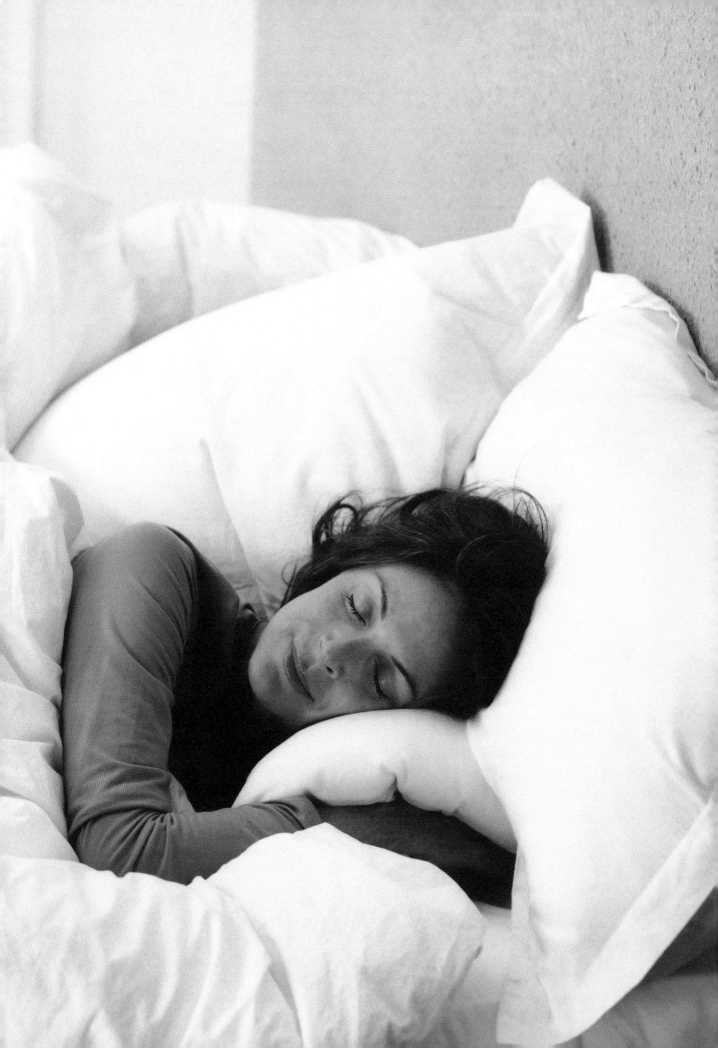

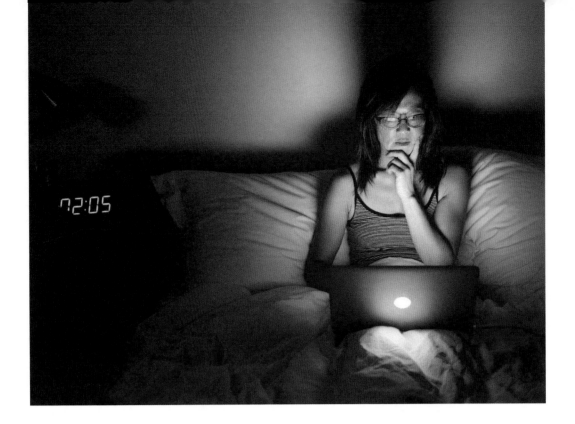

THE IMPORTANCE OF SLEEP

Getting a restless nation to sleep

BY DAVID DUDLEY

FOR MILLIONS OF US, THE PURsuit of a good night's rest has become a kind of dark obsession. We're getting an hour less sleep per night, on average, than our forebears did a few generations ago. In 1942, only 11 percent of Americans slept six hours or less a night. By 2013, 40 percent did. Older adults are more vulnerable to sleep disorders, particularly obstructive sleep apnea, an intermittent breathing problem that causes serious health issues.

> Sleep Crisis

So many seem to be getting so little shut-eye that the Centers for Disease Control and Prevention has declared the sorry state of the nation's slumber a public health problem: Some 80 million adult Americans aren't getting enough sleep, the latest CDC study says. The National Institutes of Health states that 70 million adults suffer from sleep difficulties. In a 2015 survey of the top health complaints, sleep issues have climbed to No. 2. "It didn't use to be in the top five," says Mayo Clinic pulmonologist Timothy Morgenthaler, M.D., former president of the American Academy of Sleep Medicine. "Is there a sleep crisis? Well, define 'crisis.' These problems have definitely increased radically in the past few years."

Experts have identified several reasons why, including rising obesity and the unprecedented number of adults taking medications such as antidepressants. But for many, sleeping less is a choice: We're watching TV, fiddling on Facebook or otherwise occupied in front of electronic screens deep into the wee hours. This consumes 11 hours per day for an average adult, according to Nielsen estimates. All those tablets and smartphones and TVs collectively conspire to steal our sleep by emitting a high-intensity light that scrambles our circadian rhythms, which evolved to follow the cycles of natural daylight.

We're also subject to the workplace phenomenon of "sleep shaming"—when alpha-achiever types humblebrag about how late they work and how early they rise. This is hardly new: Thomas Edison, a champion sleep shamer, claimed to need no more than four hours of rack time and demanded the same of his employees. He's a formative figure in what Penn State labor and

Sleep is the brain's overnight rinse cycle, a time for flushing cellular debris.

employee relations history professor Alan Derickson, in his book *Dangerously Sleepy*, dubbed "the cult of manly wakefulness." (A period exemplar: Charles Lindbergh, who claimed to stay up for 33 hours during his transatlantic flight.) "We are always hearing people talk about 'loss of sleep' as a calamity. They better call it loss of time," Edison once proclaimed. "There is really no reason why men should go to bed at all."

> The Sleep Gap

On the other side of this late-night culture war stand pro-sleep evangelists such as The Huffington Post founder Arianna Huffington, whose book *The Sleep Revolution* joins several new self-help tomes promising to restore sanity to the night. "We're a society that's on the clock," says Matt Berical, contributing editor of *Van Winkle's*, an online publication devoted to sleep. "The next great struggle for us is, how are we going to get rest? Sleep inequality will be a big issue in the future. There are services that will be available only to people who can afford it."

The sleep gap is just one of many stubborn disparities that haunt the night. The wealthy sleep better than the less affluent, and whites sleep better than African Americans. Women sleep more than men, although men are more satisfied with their sleep. And age itself is a factor, says University of Chicago epidemiologist Diane Lauderdale, Ph.D. "Young adults sleep better and sleep more. If you expect to be able to sleep like you did when you were 26, you're going to be disappointed."

Lauderdale goes on to caution that, when it comes to how well we're sleeping, we're not the best judges. Since population-based studies tend to rely on self-reported surveys, the current epidemic of sleep woes could in part be in our (aging) heads. "Everyone personally used to sleep better, so it sounds reasonable to think it's something the whole population is going through," she says. "The fact that we are being bombarded with people telling us we're not sleeping enough can influence our perceptions."

What isn't in dispute is how absolutely critical it is to get enough sleep. In animal studies, sleep deprivation has a horrific impact—rats kept awake died in agony within weeks. But it wasn't until UCLA biomathematician Van Savage published a 2007 paper comparing sleep duration and metabolic rates that scientists were able to mount "a compelling argument for the core function of sleep," says Charles Czeisler, chief of the Division of Sleep and Circadian Disorders at Brigham and Women's Hospital in Boston. According to the theory, sleep is the brain's overnight rinse cycle, a time for flushing cellular debris generated by metabolic activity. "The brain has to go offline during that process," Czeisler says. "That's what we call sleep."

There's no getting around the damage done by failing to run your neurochemical dishwasher: One bad night translates into a day of diminished executive function, foggy memory and sludgy mental acuity. In older adults, bad sleep may speed the development of cognitive impairments. ■

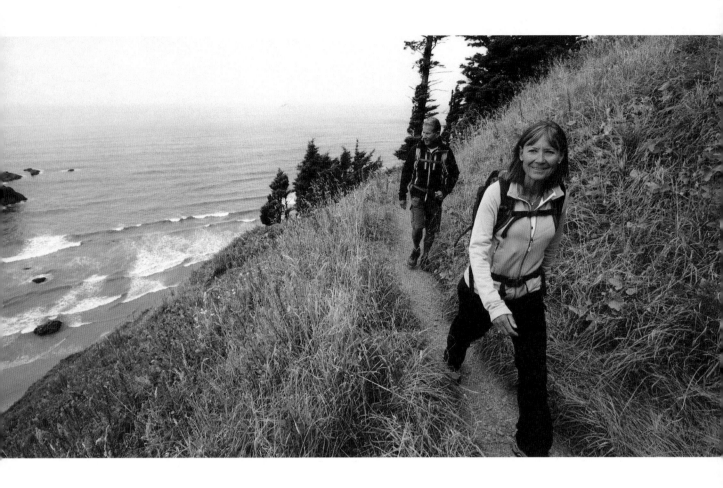

7 DAYTIME HABITS TO HELP YOU SLEEP BETTER

Exercise, a good routine and the right foods all contribute to a better night's slumber

BY JESSICA MIGALA

HOW'D YOU SLEEP LAST NIGHT? If you're like more than a third of adults, you're probably not getting the recommended seven hours a night, and it might not be for lack of trying. New research finds that what you do during the day can have just as big an impact on the quality and quantity of your sleep as what you do just before bed. Here are seven habits to start today—so you can sleep better tonight.

1 Get some green.

At least once a day, head to a local park, tend to your garden or take a scenic walk. Adults age 65 and older who spend time in nature are more likely to sleep better, according to a study from the University of Illinois at Urbana-Champaign. When you commune with nature, you're staying active and boosting your mental health—two factors that have been shown to improve sleep quality when you go to tuck in.

2 Love your routine.

Having a daily routine is far from boring—in fact, it may be vital for your well-being. Canadian research recently found that both good sleepers and insomniacs participated in activities throughout the day, but it was the good sleepers who did them at consistent times. (For example: Go to the gym in the morning, head to work, meet friends for dinner, etc.) A regular routine can help set your biological rhythms so that your body is ready for bed when you are.

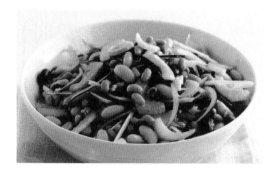

3 Load up on legumes.

If you want better zzz's, focus on eating more fiber (found in large amounts in foods like lentils and beans) and getting less saturated fat and sugar, a study in the *Journal of Clinical Sleep Medicine* suggests. That pattern of eating was related to more time spent in restorative slow-wave sleep and fewer middle-of-the-night wake-ups. And, yep, that might explain why you wake up feeling sluggish after a burger, fries and milkshake combo.

4 Work it out.

You may be reluctant to work out later in the day, worried that getting sweaty would make it too stimulating to get to sleep at night. Go right ahead: it's okay to balance to take that jog or snag a spot with a trainer in the evening, suggests research in *Sleep Medicine*. People who reported vigorous evening exercise didn't get worse sleep—97 percent said they logged just as good or better sleep on days they hit the gym compared with nonexercise days.

5 See the light.

Workers who were exposed to natural daylight through windows got 46 more minutes of sleep compared with those in windowless environments, reports a study the *Journal of Clinical Sleep Medicine*. Exposure to light during the day and darkness at night keeps your body's circadian rhythms in check (turn the page for a more detailed story on how to reset your body clock). If you spend your day in a dark building, the researchers suggest going outside for a short walk or lunch to snag some sun.

6 Stay in the moment.

Mindfulness meditation—the practice of being aware of thoughts, feelings and sensations in the moment, without judging them as "good" or "bad"—has received a lot of buzz recently, and for good reason. In a study in *JAMA Internal Medicine*, older adults who took a mindfulness class two hours a week for six weeks benefited from improved sleep quality more so than those learning healthy bedtime habits (such as how to wind down before bed). What's more, mindfulness helped reduce fatigue during the day. So next time you're walking to the train, sense your feet on the pavement or how the breeze feels on your skin.

7 Pop meds right.

Educated white women older than 50 are the most likely segment of the U.S. population to rely on sleeping pills, research from the Centers for Disease Control and Prevention shows. If you need this extra help to catch your zzz's, take them on an empty stomach. For some meds, washing them down with dinner can delay the time it takes them to work. Because the guidelines differ depending on what you're taking—over-the-counter products typically aren't affected by food—this is a reminder to always read the instructions on the medication label (or ask your pharmacist) to learn the guidelines on yours. It can mean all the difference between slipping into slumber and lying awake and staring at the ceiling. Sweet dreams. ■

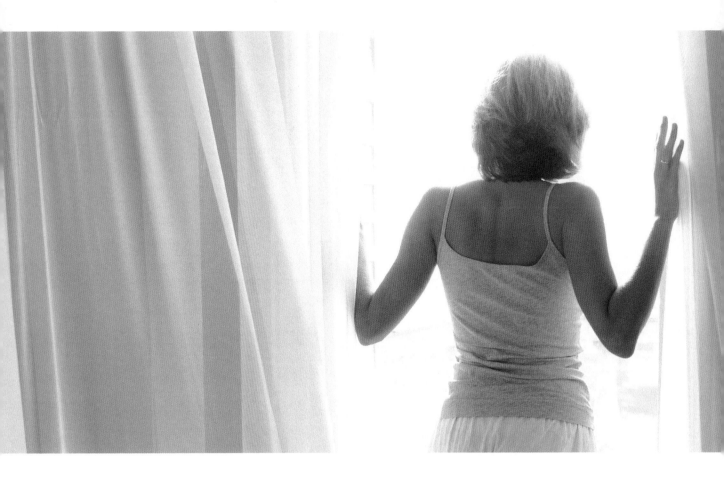

RESET YOUR BODY CLOCK FOR BETTER BRAIN HEALTH

Feeling mentally foggy? Your circadian rhythm may be out of sync

BY MICHELE COHEN MARILL

"**E**ARLY TO BED, EARLY TO RISE" may sound like sage advice, but if your circadian rhythm—aka your body clock—gets out of whack, it can make you sleepy when you should be alert and wakeful when you should be sleeping. Disrupted sleep patterns can also lead to poor memory, depression and even migraine headaches. Here are nine ways to reset your body clock.

> Step Into the Sunshine

Morning sunshine is an on-switch for your body clock and sends a strong wakening signal to your brain. Our circadian rhythm isn't exactly 24 hours—it's off by as much as half an hour—so morning light resets the clock. If you can't get outside, open the blinds and turn up the lights, advises Jeanne Duffy, Ph.D., a neuroscientist at Brigham and Women's Hospital in Boston.

> ### Go Online in the Morning

Blue light from electronic devices such as computer monitors delivers a powerful jump-start to your brain. By going online in the morning, you take advantage of your natural alertness early in the day and gain an extra mental edge. Blue light exposure proved even more powerful than caffeine in boosting reaction times on certain cognitive and motor tests, according to a 2013 Swedish study. Blue-light therapy also improved mood in a study of 89 older adults with major depression.

> ### Sync Your Schedule

Did you know there is a "best" time to memorize something (in the morning) and a different "best" time to be creative for many (late in the day)? Or that blood pressure medicine works best when taken at night—lowering your risk of stroke and protecting your brain? Fitting your daily activities around your body's natural rhythm can make you more productive and healthy.

> ### Avoid Fatty Foods

Eating too much bacon, fried chicken and pizza could make you sleepy and sluggish. Our eating patterns—and digestive system—are part of our body clock, and a high-fat diet can disrupt the rhythm. In an Australian study of 1,815 men between the ages of 35 and 80, those eating a high-fat diet reported more daytime sleepiness, regardless of body-mass index. Switching to a low-fat diet may reverse the effect.

> ### Cut Out Coffee

A coffee buzz feels good in the morning and makes you more alert, but late in the day it may overpower your body clock. Caffeine lingers in your system for eight to 14 hours. Only drink coffee in the afternoon or evening if you need to stay up late or if you are trying to reset your body clock to a later bedtime.

> ### Treat Your Cataracts

The cloudy cataracts we often get as we age may be blocking the blue light you need to signal your wake-sleep cycle—and dimming your alertness. When cataract surgery removes a yellowed lens, your circadian rhythm gets a boost. Studies show that cataract surgery has brain benefits, too, improving reaction time on cognitive tests and reducing daytime sleepiness.

> ### Dim the Lights

Darkness is your brain's off-switch. Late evening light keeps you awake—even if it's the glow from a television or electronic tablet. A few minutes of bright light at bedtime or in the middle of the night (such as turning on the bathroom light) sends the wrong signal to your brain. The American Medical Association also warns about sleep disruption from high-intensity LED street lights. Shut them out with light-blocking curtains or blinds.

> ### Consider Melatonin

The sleep-inducing hormone melatonin provides another important trigger for your body clock. As we age, we make less melatonin, and some medicines, such as beta-blockers, cut levels even further. A small bedtime dose (talk to your doctor) gives your body clock the cue it needs. But don't go overboard—large doses of the supplement may make you feel sleepy during the day. Talk to your doctor before taking melatonin.

> ### Crank Up the Wattage

If your daily rhythm is really out of whack, you need a stronger reset. Older adults are more likely to have a circadian rhythm condition called advanced sleep phase disorder, which causes very early bedtime and waking. Block light in the morning with blackout shades or drapes and keep the lights on at night between 7 and 9 p.m. You should be back on track fairly soon. ■

HEALTH CARE

ALL OF US NEED A SUPPORT system to maintain our good health. Medical care is a critical component. From preventive medicine to maintenance check-ups to surgery and palliative care, it's important to have a good relationship with a network of providers. Beyond medical appointments, many of us require a boost to our diets and medications with supplements, but it's essential to understand which will benefit us, and how to ensure that we don't introduce complications.

This section kicks off by looking at the old standard of health care: the annual physical. Many of us dutifully show up each year to be weighed, measured and analyzed, but new research is showing that it may not be necessary. We examine several myths related to the annual physical, including whether it's always a good idea (it isn't), if you need one even if you feel fine (you may), and whether it's always covered by insurance (not necessarily). We move on to look at four common

surgeries—and then explain why you should talk to your doctor about avoiding them, if possible, and suggest alternative treatments that don't require you to go under the knife.

Vaccines are generally associated with newborns and small children, but the more experienced among us need to keep up to date on our immunizations as well. We provide a checklist of shots you need to have—including flu, varicella and hepatitis—and give you the scoop on exactly what each injection will, and will not, do for your health.

Vitamins and supplements can be enormously helpful in boosting your health, but many of us become overwhelmed at the vast offerings on the market today. This section breaks down what you need for each decade, then explains how particular supplements may interact with your prescription and over-the-counter medications and should be taken with caution. Here's to your good health!

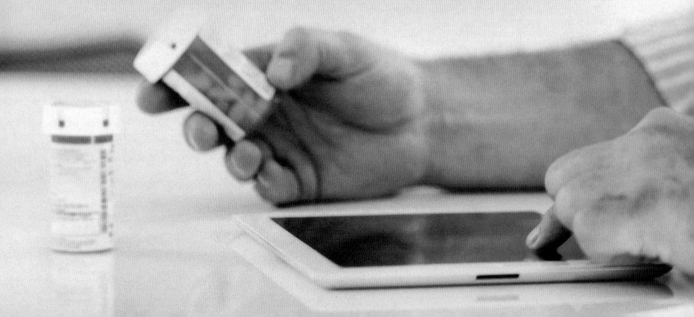

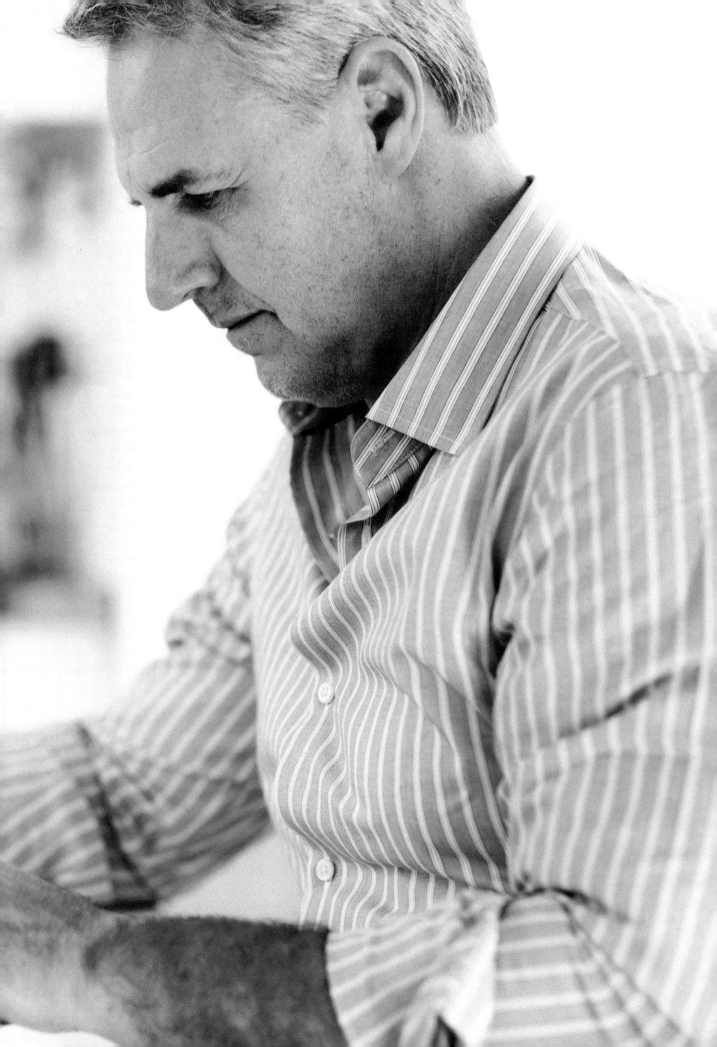

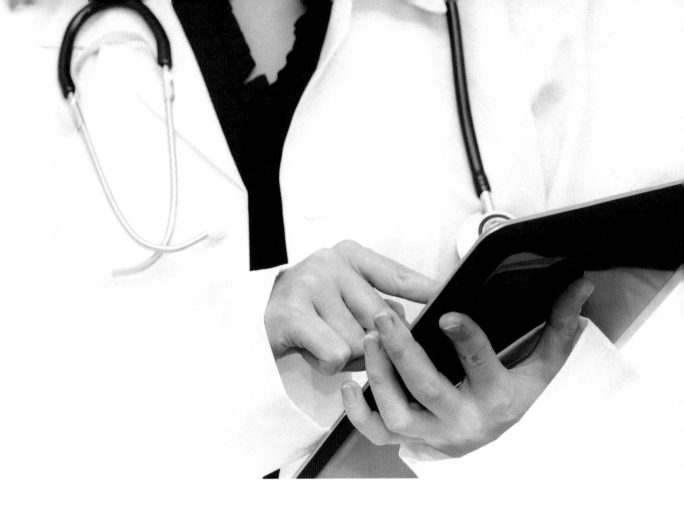

DO YOU REALLY NEED AN ANNUAL PHYSICAL?

Five myths and facts you should know about that yearly checkup

BY CANDY SAGON

THE ANNUAL PHYSICAL EXAM has been a popular fixture in American medicine since the 1940s as a way to help your doctor get to know you and your medical history, do some screening tests and maybe even catch some problems early. So you'd think that every health expert would be in favor of it. But that's just one of the myths about the annual physical—that everyone thinks it's a good idea. There are other things you should know as well, such as whether Medicare covers it. (Hint: It's complicated.)

Myth 1: An annual physical is a good idea.

Opinions are divided about whether getting checked out by your primary care doctor once a year is beneficial for those who are otherwise healthy. The majority of Americans continue to believe it is.

The *New England Journal of Medicine* featured dueling editorials by physicians for and against the annual exam. One side argued that there's no evidence that these exams help Americans stay healthier or reduce deaths, and that basically they waste time and money better spent on sicker patients. The other side disagreed, saying the exams help build a doctor-patient relationship and provide the opportunity for doctors to perform and important and thorough health review.

Myth 2: An annual exam ensures you're healthy.

Not exactly. An annual exam does give a quick snapshot of your health, but its aim is to focus on commonplace prevention and screening and to help you establish a doctor-patient relationship in case of an illness. Even the physicians who authored the editorial against an annual exam agree that a periodic checkup is important for establishing that relationship and that primary care doctors need to monitor their patients' attention to preventive care.

For example, during an annual exam a doctor should do things like discuss a patient's family medical history for increased risks of heart attack, hypertension, diabetes or cancer; listen to the heart and abdomen; measure blood pressure; and talk about the need for various screening tests like a colonoscopy at age 50 or a Pap test for women, as well as needed immunizations—all subjects that wouldn't come up during a regular doctor visit for a specific problem.

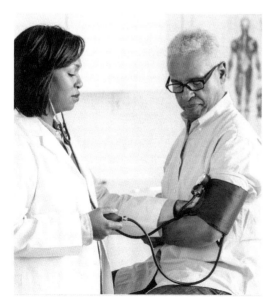

Myth 3: I feel fine. I don't need an annual physical.

Maybe you don't need an exam every year, but it's important to maintain periodic contact with your physician, especially after age 50. You may not even know you're having symptoms. Some serious conditions may not have obvious symptoms, especially in the early, more easily treatable stages—for example, high blood pressure, high cholesterol, diabetes, colon cancer and cervical cancer. A routine checkup by your doctor can include these basic screenings. Doctors can also make sure you've gotten immunizations important for older adults.

Myth 4: Medicare will cover the cost of an annual physical.

Not quite. Medicare covers two types of physical exams: a "Welcome to Medicare" exam when you first sign up, and what is called a yearly wellness visit. You have to ask the doctor's office specifically for the free Medicare wellness visit so that it gets coded correctly on the invoice. Don't just ask for a physical. If you prefer to have a physical, you'll have to pay the doctor's charge yourself unless you have a Medicare Advantage Plan or secondary insurance (such as from a former employer) that covers it. But be aware that Medicare supplemental insurance, known as Medigap, does not cover this cost.

Myth 5: If an exam is free, there's no downside.

Some think there is. For the patient, there's the time and travel to see the doctor, as well as possible "false positive" results from lab tests that could suggest a problem where there isn't one and cause you worry and additional testing. On the other hand, regular free checkups could help more people get recommended preventive services and motivate more high-risk and low-income groups to see their doctor.

So should you have have an annual physical? Best advice: Ask your doctor. ∎

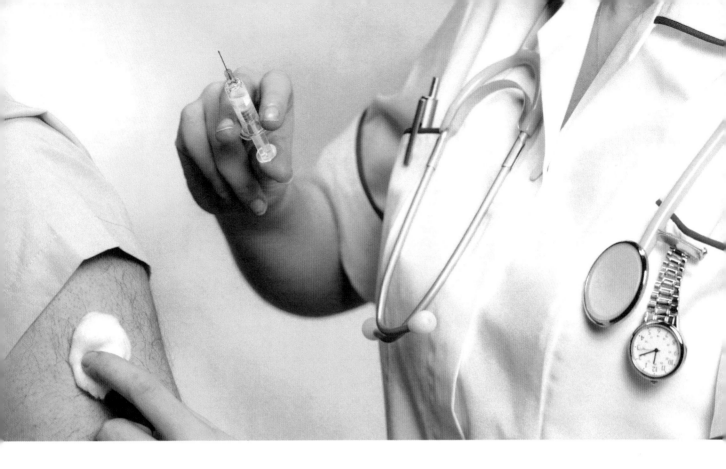

YOUR 50+ VACCINE CHECKLIST

Make sure your immunizations are up to date

CHECK WITH YOUR DOCTOR about vaccines you may need. Here are those generally recommended.

> Flu Shot

Who needs it: Everyone over 50, every year.

The lowdown: Centers for Disease Control and Prevention (CDC) research suggests that the flu shot keeps thousands of older adults out of the hospital each flu season. Researchers formulate the flu shot based on predictions about which flu viruses are most likely to land in the United States.

"Sometimes we hit it on the head; other times we miss one of the major circulating strains," says John Epling Jr., M.D., chair of family medicine at SUNY Upstate Medical University. "But getting an annual flu shot is one of the best ways we have to prevent flu." Most insurance plans cover the flu shot, or can direct you to a location where the cost is low. If you get your shot at a pharmacy or community clinic, be sure to notify your doctor's office (you can send a copy of the receipt) so they can add it to your records, Epling says.

> Hepatitis A

Who needs it: Anyone with liver disease. Otherwise, ask your doctor.

The lowdown: When people with liver disease contract hepatitis A, they have longer hospital stays than people without underlying liver trouble, according to recent research published in Hepatology. This disease can be spread through food and is more common in developing countries. Check cdc.gov/travel/destinations/list before you head to another country—this vaccine might be recommended.

> Hepatitis B

Who needs it: Anyone with HIV, kidney disease, diabetes or chronic liver disease. Otherwise, ask your doctor.

The lowdown: Many people with liver disease fail to get this shot, says Jonathan Temte, M.D., a professor of family medicine and community health at the University of Wisconsin, and that's a problem. Hepatitis can wreak havoc on your liver, and if you already have liver issues, it can be even worse.

> Herpes Zoster (Shingles)

Who needs it: Everyone 60 and older, unless you have a weakened immune system or HIV.

The lowdown: Shingles can be "excruciatingly painful," Temte says. However, only about 28 percent of people over 60 are immunized against it, according to CDC estimates. One reason: The shot's price tag, which often ranges around $200. "I've been struck in practice by the number of my patients who know about this vaccine but decline to receive it because they know also it's a very expensive vaccine, and they just can't afford it," Temte says. Pay out of pocket if you can, but if not, check out Merck's Patient Assistance Program at merckhelps.com/zostavax.

> Hib

Who needs it: Anyone with asplenia (the absence of normal spleen function) or sickle cell disease or who's had a hematopoietic stem cell transplant. Otherwise, ask your doctor.

The lowdown: This shot protects against Haemophilus influenzae type B, a serious bacterial disease that can strike older people with certain medical conditions.

> Meningococcal

Who needs it: Everyone with asplenia. Otherwise, ask your doctor.

The lowdown: This shot protects you against forms of meningitis that, while not common, can be deadly.

> Pneumococcal PCV13 and PPSV23

Who needs it: People 65 and over—but tell your doctor if you if you smoke or have heart disease, lung disease, alcoholism, diabetes or chronic liver disease. The shot is also recommended for some people younger than 65. Tell your doctor if you are pregnant, have a weakened immune system, HIV, kidney disease or poor kidney function, asplenia (the absence of normal spleen function), heart disease, lung disease, alcoholism, diabetes or chronic liver disease.

The lowdown: The doses are usually given two to 12 months apart—ask your doctor what's best for you. These shots can reduce your chances of potentially deadly pneumonia and bloodstream infections. "The older we get, the more our immune system fails to protect us, so the vaccine will provide added protection," Temte says.

> Td/Tdap

Who needs it: Adults generally need a booster every 10 years.

The lowdown: Before 2005, this shot just protected you from tetanus and diphtheria. Now, it also shields you from pertussis. Your grandkids will thank you for taking this shot: Pertussis causes an upper respiratory infection that tends to be self-limited in adults, but in kids it causes whooping cough, which can be a serious deadly disease at times, especially for young kids before their first immunization before two months.

> Varicella (chicken pox)

Who needs it: Anyone who didn't have the disease as a child—unless you have HIV or a weakened immune system.

The lowdown: Two doses will give you about 90 percent protection against chicken pox.

> One More Thing

If you're traveling outside the country, check with the CDC to see if you need any vaccines. Some potentially deadly diseases can be prevented if you get innoculated before you go to the areas that incubate them. ■

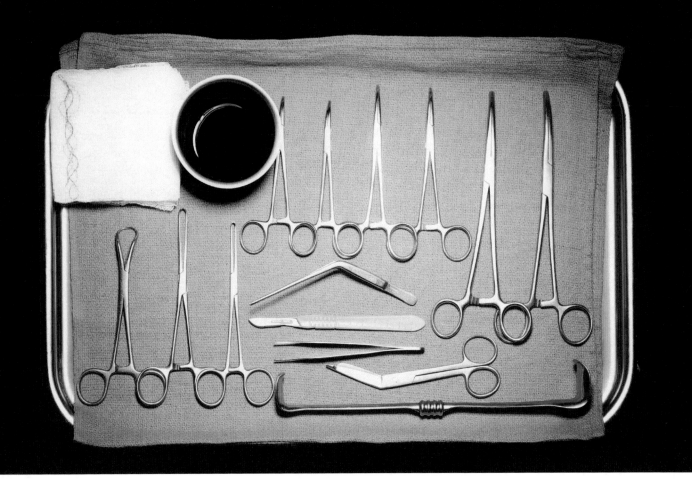

4 SURGERIES YOU MAY BE ABLE TO AVOID

Reasons to think twice before going under the knife

BY KAREN CHENEY

ANY SURGERY IS DANGEROUS. Even some minor procedures come with major risks, such as bleeding, blood clots, infections and damage to other organs.

The four operations discussed on the following pages are overperformed for a variety of reasons: Some are moneymakers for hospitals and doctors, others are expedient, and still others seem to work, at least in the short term. But evidence shows that all have questionable long-term outcomes for treating certain conditions, and some may even cause harm. Here are some factors to consider with your doctor.

1 Stents for Stable Angina

Stents are tiny mesh tubes that surgeons use to prop open arteries carrying blood to the heart. If a patient is having a heart attack, a stent can be a lifesaver. But for heart disease patients with stable angina—chest pain brought on by exertion or stress—a stent is not better at preventing a heart attack or prolonging survival than lifestyle changes such as exercising and taking statins to lower cholesterol, according to a Department of Veterans Affairs study.

More than 500,000 are implanted each year for stable chest pain, says Sanjay Kaul, M.D., a cardiologist at Cedars-Sinai Medical Center

The four operations discussed on the following pages are overperformed for a variety of reasons: Some are money-makers for hospitals and doctors, others are expedient, and still others seem to work, at least in the short term.

in Los Angeles. Surgeons frequently insert the stents during heart-catheterization procedures to evaluate patients' blood vessels, says Lee Lucas, Ph.D., an epidemiologist at Maine Medical Center Research Institute, who argues that the catheterization should be done first as a diagnostic test, and stenting done later, if necessary. "This should be a two-stage procedure, but patients never get to leave the cath lab to think about it," says Lucas.

> **Alternatives to Surgery**
If your doctor orders a heart catheterization, ask that he or she wait to perform any treatment such as stenting in a separate procedure. Even before submitting to a heart cath, make sure you've explored other alternatives. Have you had a stress test? Do you adhere to a strict diet, exercise, or take medications to manage your cholesterol? "The reality is that 20 percent of patients who undergo this [catheterization with stents] do not have any symptoms, 30 to 50 percent have not had a stress test, and 30 percent are not treated with medical therapy first," says Kaul. If plaque is forming in your arteries, this is a systemic disease; a stent won't keep even a full inch of your arteries clear. You'll still need aggressive medical therapy to prevent future problems.

2 Complex Spinal Fusion for Stenosis

With spinal fusion, a surgeon places bone grafts that "weld" two or more vertebrae together to prevent motion and stop pain. The procedure is often used to treat back pain from spinal stenosis, which occurs when the soft tissues between the vertebrae flatten out, creating pressure on the spinal cord or nerves that go to the back, arms, neck, shoulders and legs. There is little consensus on how best to relieve pain from stenosis, so doctors tend to develop their own preferences, says Richard Deyo, M.D., professor of medicine at Oregon Health & Science University.

Their top treatment choice increasingly seems to be fusion. Deyo recently studied the records of more than 30,000 Medicare patients who underwent surgery for stenosis of the lower back and found that complex fusion procedures (in which surgeons place bone grafts between multiple vertebrae) had increased an astounding fifteen-fold between 2002 and 2007.

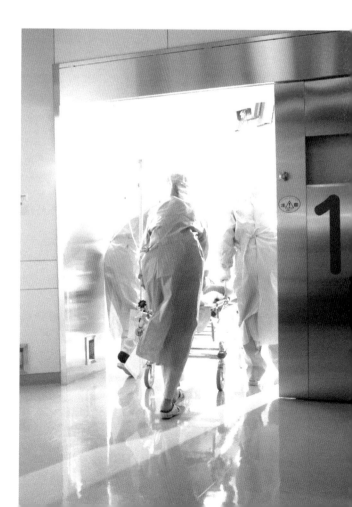

The risks are significant: Those who underwent complex fusion were nearly three times more likely to suffer life-threatening complications than those who underwent less invasive surgery. Previous studies have also found that most fusion patients experience no more relief from their chronic back pain than those who had physical and behavioral therapy. "There is even some evidence that [complex fusion surgery] is worse than other surgeries," says Floyd J. Fowler Jr., Ph.D., senior scientific advisor for the Informed Medical Decisions Foundation. "The vertebrae right above and below the fusion have to do a lot more bending, and it puts stress on your back above and below."

> Alternatives to Surgery

Before considering any type of back surgery, make sure you have exhausted more conservative measures, including physical therapy, cortisone injections, acupuncture and medications. "Probably less than 5 percent of all back pain requires surgery," says Arnold Weil, M.D., clinical assistant professor of rehabilitation medicine at Emory University School of Medicine in Atlanta.

3 Hysterectomy for Uterine Fibroids

Each year approximately 600,000 American women have hysterectomies, or removal of the uterus, and studies show that the vast majority are unnecessary. A hysterectomy is critical when the patient has cancer (which is the case for about 10 percent of those women). But most patients undergo the procedure for quality-of-life concerns such as heavy bleeding or pain caused by uterine fibroids— typically benign growths in the uterine wall.

Complications are common. Women who undergo a hysterectomy have a 60 percent increased risk of incontinence by age 60, a University of California, San Francisco study found. A hysterectomy that includes removal of the ovaries—an oophorectomy—throws the patient into instant menopause, which can have a host of side effects and complications in and of itself. These patients also face a higher risk of heart disease and lung cancer, says William Parker, M.D., coauthor of *A Gynecologist's Second Opinion* and lead investigator of a study on the long-term health consequences of hysterectomy.

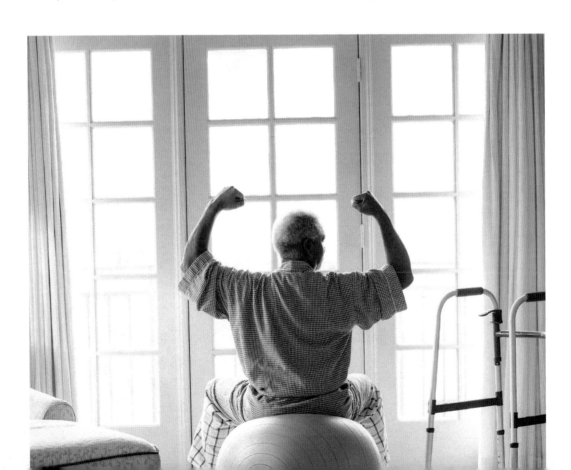

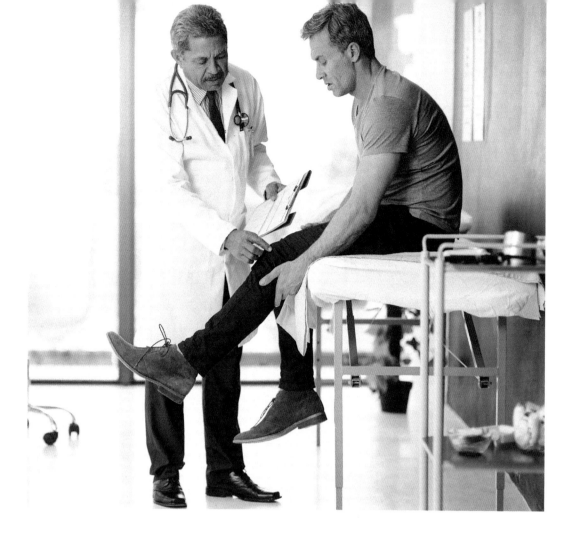

> Alternatives to Surgery

If you suffer from uterine fibroids, ask your doctor about other options, including uterine-artery embolization, in which the arteries leading to the uterus are blocked, causing the fibroids to stop growing. You might also consider a new procedure, focused ultrasound, which shrinks fibroids via ultrasound waves. "It's kind of amazing that we've had all these alternative procedures for many years and they haven't gained a lot of traction," says Parker.

4 Knee Arthroscopy for Osteoarthritis

With this procedure a surgeon places a tiny camera in the knee, then inserts small instruments through other incisions to repair torn or aging cartilage. Studies show the operation can work when patients have in fact torn their meniscal tissue, but it is no more successful than noninvasive remedies in treating osteoarthritis of the knee. In one study, 178 patients with osteoarthritis

received either physical and medical therapy without surgery, or therapy plus surgery. After two years the two groups had nearly identical outcomes, reporting less pain and stiffness and more mobility.

> Alternatives to Surgery

If you have knee pain, "start with the least harmful and invasive treatment and work your way up the ladder," says Colin Nelson, editorial director of the University of Washington Medicine Health Sports and Safety Institute. This includes lifestyle changes such as exercise, as well as medication and cortisone injections. ∎

Before considering any type of back surgery, make sure you have exhausted more conservative measures.

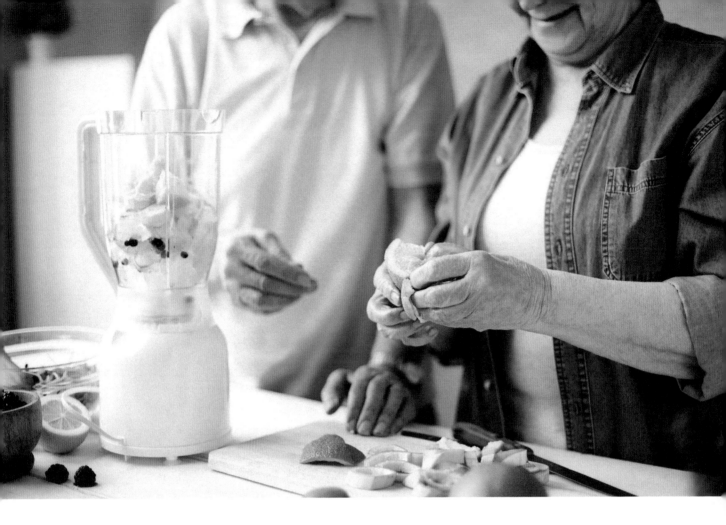

GETTING THE NUTRIENTS YOU NEED

Get an edge over osteoporosis, heart disease, even cancer

BY AMY PATUREL

I N AN IDEAL WORLD YOU WOULD get all of your nutrients from fruits, vegetables and other unprocessed whole foods. But as you enter your 50s, hormonal changes make hitting your target quotas for certain vitamins and minerals increasingly difficult. While science can't re-create everything nature has perfectly packed into whole foods, supplementing your diet with these key nutrients should help you stay on top of your game.

Dietary requirements change as you get older, so be sure that you are amending your diet and adjusting your supplements accordingly. In addition, don't start shopping before getting medical advice: Consult with your doctor before adding any of these supplements into your daily regimen.

IN YOUR 50S

> **Vitamin D and calcium** Bone loss accelerates during your 50s, especially among women. Recommended dose: 600 international units of vitamin D plus 1,000 milligrams (mg) of calcium for men and 1,200 mg for women, split into two daily doses. Good food sources: salmon, tuna, mackerel, beef liver, cheese, egg yolks are rich in vitamin D. To boost your calcium intake, eat cheese, yogurt, milk, figs.

> **Omega-3 fatty acids** Omega-3s help reduce plaque buildup in the arteries and inhibit inflammation. Omega-3s are important for reducing inflammation wherever it comes up, whether as heart disease, cancer or Alzheimer's. Recommended dose: 1,000 mg of EPA and DHA omega-3s per day. Good food sources: flaxseed oil, salmon, walnuts, edamame.

> **Probiotics** The older you are, the more vulnerable your system is to unhealthy bacteria. Probiotics help by reintroducing good bacteria. Recommended dose: 1 billion to 10 billion CFUs a few days a week. Good food sources: yogurt, kefir, kimchi.

IN YOUR 60S

> **Vitamin B12** Even a mild vitamin B12 deficiency may put older adults at risk for dementia. But stomach acid, which is required for the body to absorb vitamin B12 from food, begins to decline during your 50s, so the Institute of Medicine recommends getting your B12 levels checked and supplement if necessary. Recommended dose: 2.4 micrograms daily. Good food sources: clams, beef liver, trout, cheeseburger, sirloin.

> **Omega-3s** DHA is the most abundant omega-3 fatty acid in the brain's cell membranes. Over the past decade, studies have linked omega-3 fatty acids to brain benefits ranging from better blood flow and increased health of brain cells to improved mood and enhanced memory. Unfortunately, as you age, your brain cells gradually lose the ability to absorb DHA, starving your mind and compromising both brain function and memory retention. Recommended dose: 1,000 milligrams of DHA and EPA per day. Good food sources: flaxseed oil, salmon, walnuts, edamame.

> **Vitamin D** For years, scientists thought vitamin D's only role was to enhance the absorption of calcium from food. Now research shows that vitamin D can reduce chronic pain, guard against heart disease, even potentially ward off cancer. The ideal source of this critical nutrient is sunlight. But your body's ability to synthesize vitamin D from sunlight declines as you age. Recommended dose: 600 international units daily. Look for supplements that contain vitamin D3, an active form that's more effective than its vitamin D2 counterpart. Good food sources even potentially help ward off cancer: salmon, tuna, mackerel, beef liver, cheese, egg yolks.

IN YOUR 70S

> **Vitamin B12** See In Your 60s.   > **Vitamin D** See In Your 60s.

> **Protein** When you hit your 70s, your ability to build muscle mass deteriorates. Plus, your protein needs grow even as your intake and appetite may wane. Once you lose more than 10 percent of your muscle mass, your immune system doesn't function properly. The good news: Supplementing with protein powders or pills can increase lean body mass and muscle. Recommended dose: 20 to 30 grams of whey protein powder mixed into a daily shake. Good food sources: beef, chicken, beans, almonds.

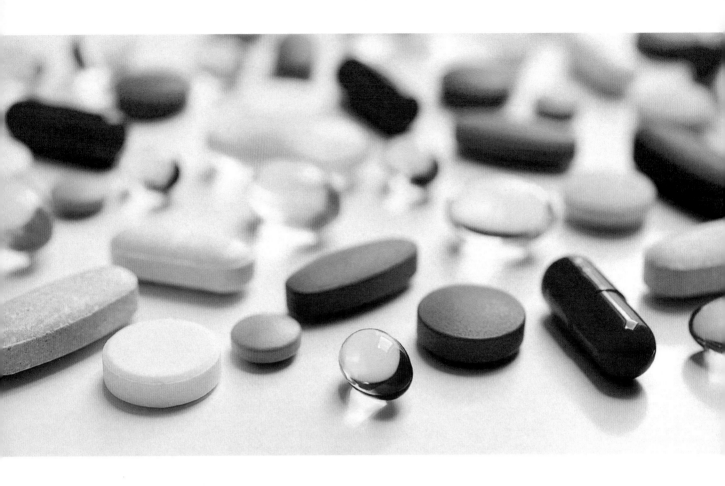

SWALLOW WITH CARE

Some health remedies may trigger dangerous reactions with your medications

BY ELAINE K. HOWLEY

MANY AMERICANS CONCEDE they have too many pills already, and yet they keep adding dietary and herbal supplements to their home pharmacies. Dima Qato, Ph.D., assistant professor at the University of Chicago, Illinois, School of Pharmacy, led one 2016 study that found more than two-thirds of adults ages 62 to 85 take at least five medications—prescription drugs, over-the-counter medications or dietary supplements. Some supplements or over-the-counter medications can make prescription drugs less effective or boost dangerous side effects.

Virtually everything you ingest—food, supplements and medications—has the potential to interact with something else. Most of us probably don't realize there could be any danger, but supplements are not regulated like prescription drugs. Tell your doctor or pharmacist about every supplement or over-the-counter drug you use regularly.

> Fish Oil

The omega-3 fatty acids found in fish oil have long been hailed as heart healthy. Yet for some people, fish oil capsules can elevate the risk of excessive bleeding when combined with a common anti-coagulant, warfarin, sold under the brand names Coumadin and Jantoven.

> Ginkgo Biloba Supplements

As with fish oil, taking ginkgo biloba supplements while on warfarin may raise your risk of internal bleeding. Manufacturers tout the product's ability to support memory and cognitive function by increasing blood flow in the brain.

> St. John's Wort

If you're taking an antidepressant but still feeling low, resist the temptation to add a little St. John's wort to your daily regimen. This is an herbal supplement taken to treat mild depression, but mixing it with selective serotonin reuptake inhibitors (SSRIs) may cause a dangerous condition called serotonin syndrome. Serotonin syndrome can cause diarrhea and shivering in its milder forms, but it can escalate to mental confusion, fever and seizures, and can even prove fatal.

> Vitamin D Supplements

Excess vitamin D can cause issues for patients taking thiazide diuretics—drugs that include hydrochlorothiazide (HCTZ), chlorothiazide, chlorthalidone, indapamide and metolazone, which are used to treat hypertension and edema—and may lead to high calcium levels and kidney stones, weak bones and cognitive problems.

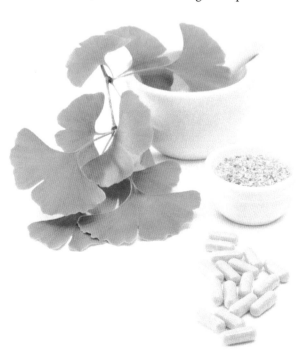

> NSAIDs

These drugs are so ubiquitous, we seldom stop to think before taking a tablet or two at the first sign of a headache. But this could be dangerous for patients who are also taking antidepressants. Mixing NSAIDs with any class of antidepressant can increase your risk of intracranial hemorrhage (bleeding inside the skull). In some people, this type of bleeding can lead to permanent brain damage and death.

> Erectile Dysfunction Supplements

ED supplements may be billed as all natural, but some of their active ingredients could pose risks combined with nitrates, prescribed for angina (chest pain tied to coronary artery disease). In one study more than 80 percent carry traces of PDE5Is, the active ingredient in drugs like Viagra and Cialis. Ads already caution not to mix the drugs with nitrates, or you risk a potentially fatal drop in blood pressure.

> Coenzyme Q10 Supplements

If you're taking a statin to lower cholesterol, you may have been told to take a CoQ10 supplement to offset related muscle pain and weakness. But if you're also taking a medication to lower blood pressure, be careful. CoQ10 supplements may interact by further lowering blood pressure. CoQ10 also reduces blood sugar levels, so if you have diabetes or low blood sugar, you'll have to watch your sugars carefully and adjust your insulin or glucose intake. Lastly, this supplement may interact with blood thinners, so talk with your doctor before adding it if you take warfarin or a daily aspirin.

> Niacin Supplements

Niacin helps the body convert food into fuel. People who also take cholesterol-lowering statins should consult with their doctor before taking it. Niacin in combination with these drugs may cause liver damage and muscle inflammation. Diabetics should also beware because niacin may increase blood sugar levels, disrupting the efficacy of insulin. ■

MIND, BODY AND SPIRIT

THERE ARE A LOT OF PRAC-tices, remedies and tricks out there to help you boost your overall health even more. We tend to think of odd-looking exercises and treatments as fads, or consign them to the young. But in fact, many of these so-called "new" health offerings are rooted in ancient traditions and are proven methods of healing. Yoga and tai chi can provide physical relief for many maladies and offer wonderful benefits for the mind.

Yoga has been a hot trend for years now, but in the age of Instagram it's easy to be put off by photos of yogis balancing on one arm. Yoga is actually an ancient healing practice that is open to everyone: it can help you increase strength and flexibility, calm your mind and increase your overall energy. We offer suggestions for easing into a practice that is just right for you.

Tai chi is another mind-body exercise that provides similar benefits to yoga and may sharpen cognition and reduce anxiety and depression. Meditation, or mindfulness, is the practice of observing and accepting our thoughts as they occur without judging or attempting to change them. A regular meditation practice, even just ten minutes a day, can greatly reduce stress and improve overall health (and it is guaranteed to be injury free).

We wrap up by examining gadgets and devices that can bump up your health, from monitoring your fitness to organizing your pills, and present a fascinating case study on the citizens of Nagano, Japan, who have an incredibly long life span (and might have some advice we can use). In short, everything in this section is optional, but it could mean the difference between feeling good and being your absolute best.

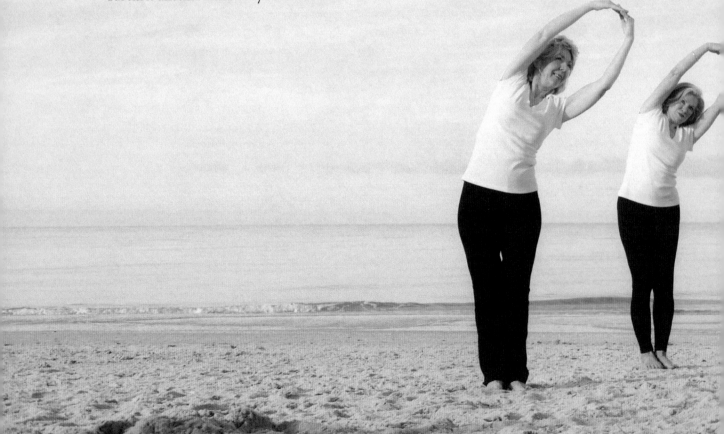

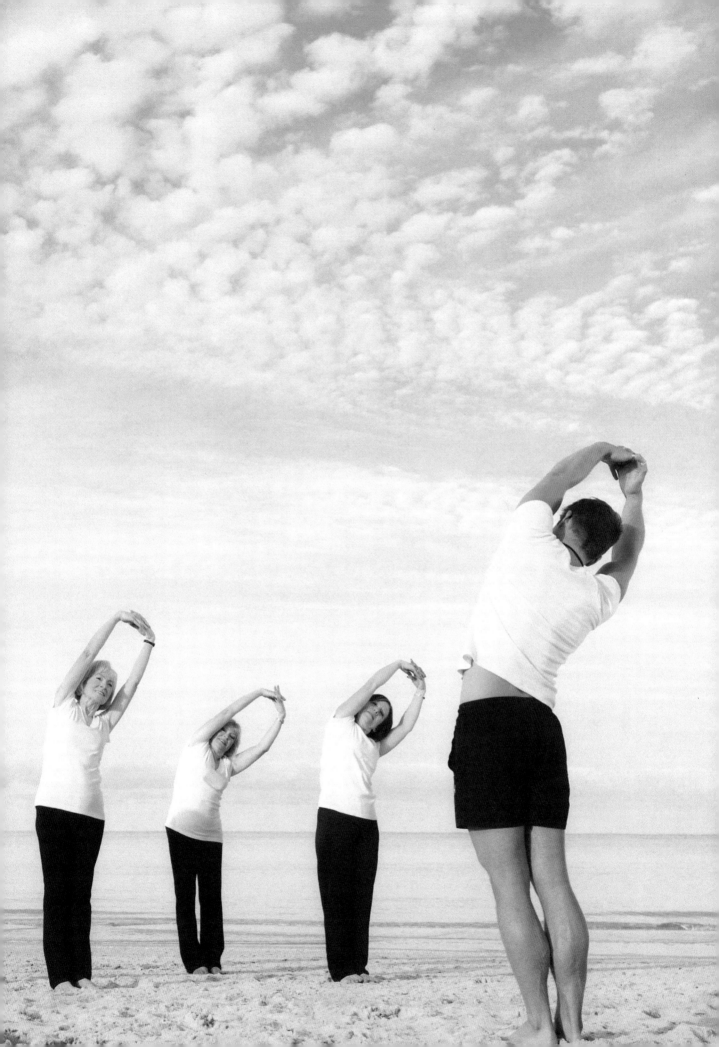

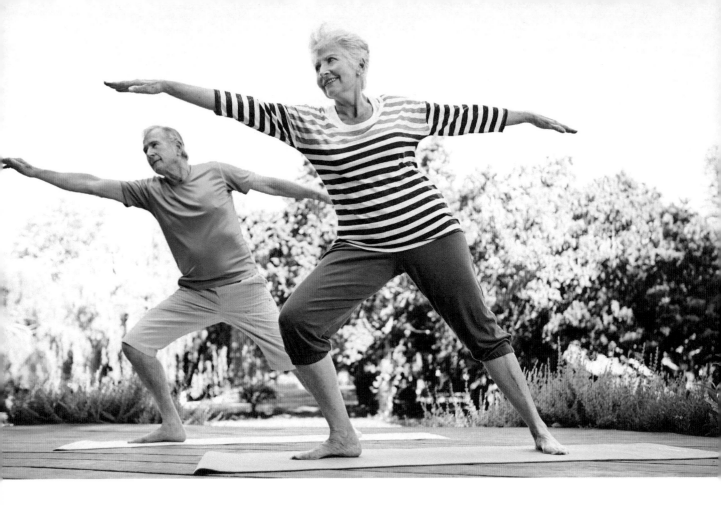

7 WAYS TO EASE INTO YOGA

An expert's guide on how to get started

BY CAROL KRUCOFF

HAVE YOU RESOLVED TO EX-ercise and get healthier in the near future? Health and medical experts say you might want to try yoga. In fact, a Harris Interactive poll of a cross section of 5,000 Americans found that 6.1 percent—which translated to nearly 14 million adults—say their doctor or therapist recommended yoga to them.

Yoga is an ancient healing practice that has become increasingly popular in our modern, stressful world as a powerful way to stretch and strengthen the body, relax and calm the mind, enhance energy and lift the spirit. Doctors often recommend yoga to people over 50 because it can help lower blood pressure, ease pain and improve balance. But people stick with the ancient practice because they find it improves their mood, reduces stress and, simply put, makes them happier.

Unfortunately, many yoga instructors are not trained to adapt the practice to older bodies. And America's booming interest in yoga has led to an increase in classes that are called yoga, but are actually "yoga-flavored" exercise classes taught by instructors whose yoga training may be limited to a weekend workshop. Unless a yoga teacher creates a safe class designed for older adults, this practice meant to heal may cause harm. To safely reap the many benefits of yoga, it's important to understand these seven essential yoga facts:

1 Yoga can be good medicine.

When new students come to my yoga class, I typically ask them what they're seeking from the practice. "Flexibility" and "stress reduction" are the most common answers, since most people associate yoga with stretching and relaxation. But that's changed in recent years, as a growing body of scientific evidence suggests that yoga offers many other health benefits, including reducing high blood pressure, relieving back pain and improving sleep. Now when I ask new students why they've come to yoga, more and more people tell me that it's just what their doctor ordered. A strong part of this yoga-as-medicine trend is fueled by people over age 50, who represent the most diverse mix of abilities of any age group.

> Now when I ask new students why they've come to yoga, more and more people tell me that it's just what their doctor ordered.

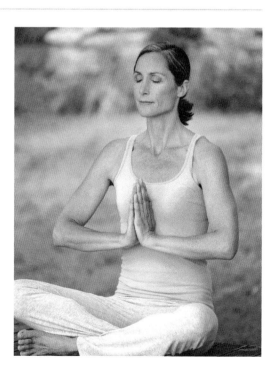

2 Yoga is not just for the fit and flexible.

Saying that you're not flexible enough to practice yoga is like thinking that your house is too messy to hire a maid. The idea that you must twist yourself into a pretzel to do yoga is one of many common misconceptions. I've taught yoga to people with a wide array of health conditions, including heart failure, osteoporosis, arthritis, fibromyalgia and back pain. The only requirement for practicing yoga is the ability to breathe.

3 You don't have to stand on your head.

While some people over 50 are extremely healthy and able to do headstands and other challenging yoga postures, much more common are older adults who fit the profile of the "average" senior in America—85 percent of whom have at least one chronic health condition and 60 percent of whom have at least two. Many also face other health challenges, such as artificial joints or prosthetic heart valves. That's why it's essential for older adults beginning yoga to find an appropriate class with an experienced and well-qualified instructor.

4 There are many styles of yoga— from "hot" to gentle.

For example, ashtanga yoga is very athletic, while kripalu yoga tends to be gentler and viniyoga is often done one-on-one in a therapeutic setting. If you attend a class that is too demanding for your specific level of fitness, you may risk injury. Be sure you're in a class that is appropriate for you, and inform the teacher of any health concerns or challenges you face. Older adults, particularly those who have been inactive, should look for a class called Gentle Yoga or one specifically geared to seniors.

5 Yoga should never hurt.

The yogic approach is very different from the Western exercise mentality of "go for the burn." Ancient texts on yoga say that a posture should be "steady and comfortable" or, according to some translations, "relaxed and stable" or "sweet and calm." So if you're straining to push yourself into a posture suitable for a magazine cover, that's gymnastics or calisthenics but not yoga. Yoga invites you to move into each posture only to the point where you feel a sensation of pleasant stretch, then allow your breath to help the pose deepen and unfold. If it hurts—back off!

6 Yoga is not just a workout.

Yoga is a powerful form of mind-body medicine that approaches health in a holistic manner, recognizing that physical ailments also have emotional and spiritual components. In one small study, researchers at Boston University School of Medicine found yoga was better than walking to improve people's moods. The tools of yoga are postures, breathing practices and meditation, which work together to balance and integrate mind, body and spirit.

7 Ask for help for a smooth start.

Consult your doctor for specific recommendations—especially if you have heart disease or any chronic health condition, if you've had surgery or if you are taking medications. Tell your doctor that you're planning to take yoga and ask for guidance, particularly about any specific movements or positions you should avoid. People with osteoporosis, for example, should usually avoid certain movements that can cause fracture—including bending forward from the waist and twisting the spine to a point of strain—which are taught in many classes. Responsible yoga teachers will ask you about your health and may seek your permission to work with your physician to create a yoga practice for you. ■

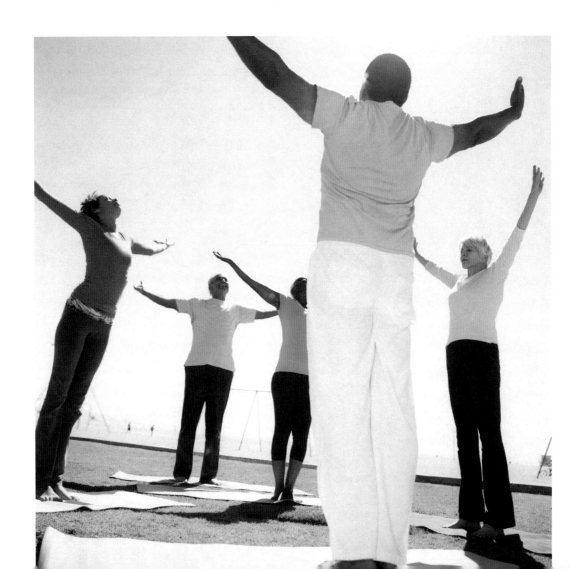

TAI CHI MAY BOOST MEMORY, THINKING SKILLS

An ancient slow-moving exercise is getting high grades

BY JANICE LLOYD

PARTICIPANTS STAND, MOVE gently and focus on their breathing while doing tai chi, a centuries-old Chinese practice. While previous studies have looked at how tai chi helps improve well-being and prevents falls among older people, ongoing studies are exploring whether it improves cognition and cardiovascular and mental health.

In a 2012 study of 120 elderly Chinese people, participants who did tai chi for 40 weeks as well as those who engaged in stimulating discussion outperformed walkers on several cognitive tests. They also showed increases in brain size and scored higher on memory and thinking tests than participants who walked or did nothing.

"You really can't go wrong with tai chi or any of the mind-body activities because they help reduce stress and build resilience," says Helen Lavretsky, M.D., a psychiatry professor at the University of California, Los Angeles, and director of the school's Late-Life Mood, Stress and Wellness Program. While Lavretsky was not involved in the study, she has conducted multiple studies to see if tai chi, yoga and meditation can lessen symptoms of depression and stress and improve cognition.

Nearly two-thirds of older people who suffer from depression do not respond to initial pharmaceutical interventions, she said. Depression weakens decision-making and attention, and it is a risk factor for Alzheimer's disease.

In a study of 112 adults age 60 and over who suffered from major depression, tai chi helped.

Seventy-three who were able to tolerate an antidepressant but had not recovered continued to take it and were assigned to 10 weeks (two hours per week) of tai chi or health education. All participants were tested for depression, anxiety, cognition, inflammation, resilience and health-related quality of life at the start of the study and afterward. Those who performed the tai chi exercises showed a greater reduction of depressive symptoms and improved cognition and decreased inflammation.

Lavretsky notes that depression can begin after people stop being mobile and no longer enjoy walking. Tai chi is a great alternative. "If you have any balance issues, start slowly and increase your agility," she said. ■

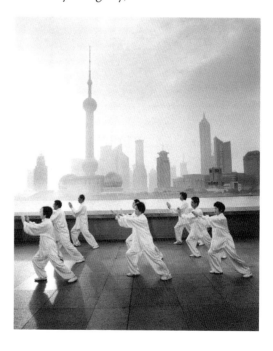

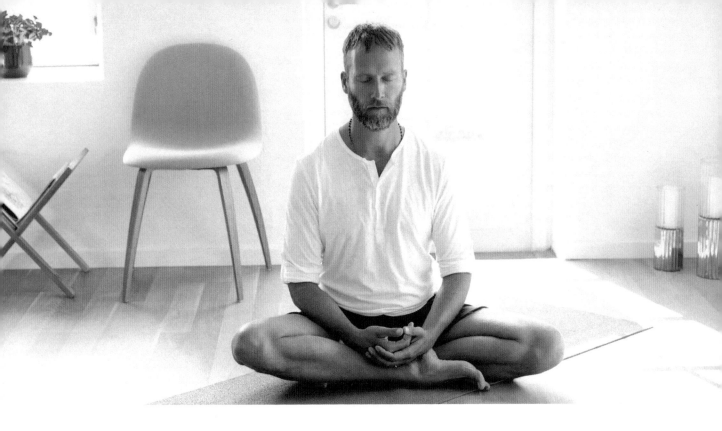

THE MEDITATION CURE

Quiet reflection is good for your brain and can lead to better choices

BY BILL STUMP

I HAD NEVER GIVEN MUCH THOUGHT to the thickness of my cerebral cortex or the volume of my brain, nor had I considered how increasing them would help regulate my attention span and emotions. But this, experts tell us, is what can happen when we meditate regularly. It's the science behind the fad that makes mindfulness—observing and accepting our thoughts as they occur in the present moment without judgment—an antidote to our ADHD way of life. It's why seemingly everyone you meet has tried meditating or plans to.

I'm one of millions—or, one of "them," as a coworker put it—who meditates daily. Even without a brain scan, I can tell you that since I've

begun, my brain is healthier. A recent checkup also indicates that my cholesterol, blood pressure, resting heart rate and a half-dozen other health metrics are at their all-time best. Studies tell me that meditation has something to do with this as well.

But the numerical aspect of my well-being is much less important to me than how I feel, and my life has been undeniably richer. I feel unhurried, sharp, focused, patient and more at ease with others and myself than I can remember. Friends have even commented on my social media postings, asking if my account has been hacked by some Russian gang that posts pictures of dogs, roses, kids and sunsets with nefarious intent. But nope, it's just me.

To be clear, I'm not an ashram-y guy. I don't burn incense, wear hemp or quote the Upanishads. I have not had a blinding moment of enlightenment. I spent much of my adult life like most everyone, building a career and raising a family. But over time, life gets complicated, and it's easy to get swept up by daily hassles and the tidal wave of hormones—cortisol, adrenaline and norepinephrine—that make us frantic, reactionary and overly sensitive.

> The numerical aspect of my well-being is much less important to me than how I feel, and my life has been undeniably richer.

For me, that meant that I became, at times, "that guy." The impatient one in the Starbucks line talking about work on my phone like I was negotiating a NATO treaty; the coach in youth soccer who told a kindly, annoying ref named George to go &%$* himself; the distracted father and husband who monitored his email as if it were the Nikkei. The things we sacrifice when we react our way through life are significant, and I knew I needed change. In search of clarity, I began to meditate. I started slowly, a few days a week, 10 minutes at a time. Today, a year later, I meditate most days for 20 minutes.

It's not mysterious. I simply sit flat-footed in a straight-backed chair and take five deep breaths—in through the nose, out through the mouth—to get started. I mentally scan my body for tension or discomfort and then continue to breathe steadily through my nose, counting breaths to keep focused on the rise and fall, not on my runaway thoughts.

When my mind wanders—and it always does—I simply note it and return to my breath.

At the end, I give myself permission to think of anything, anything at all, and my mind paradoxically goes blank for 20 or more seconds. Blissfully blank.

Even with a hundred hours of meditation behind me, I continue to marvel at how busy my mind can be, but I am even more amazed that I can climb outside my thoughts—that they don't define me but are rather "like traffic on the road" in front of me, as one guided meditation said. I find that my emotions no longer drag me around like a dog on a leash.

Meditation has worked for me, but on the rare occasions when I talk about it, I find myself focusing on the one result I haven't read or heard much about. Sitting in silence, aware of my thoughts, has lengthened the space of time between a stimulus—a thought provoked by something I see or hear—and my reaction to it.

Until I began my meditation practice, I hadn't realized that this space existed and that what I did with it determined so much in my life. That sliver of time between a comment from a friend or spouse, or getting cut off in traffic, and my reaction to it is where opportunity lies. Through practice, I'm aware that I can choose whether to take a comment personally and react in kind, or take a moment and respond more thoughtfully.

It's not easy. The space between is not filled with silence that lets you think but with a rush of clanging emotions, regrets, longing and fear—learned reactions that often move us to act based on past patterns or simple frustration. When I meditate regularly, I find that in these moments I can let all of this noise simply fall away, like silt to the bottom of a lake. This leaves me with the ability to see each unique situation clearly, to choose my reaction.

Since I've been meditating, I find that I increasingly choose wisely and that life is simpler when I do—and, apparently, healthier. So don't let what you see and read fool you. Meditation is not one thing to all people. It's not a quick fix or a simple cure for stresses large and small. It's a way to be more aware of the choices we all have each day. ∎

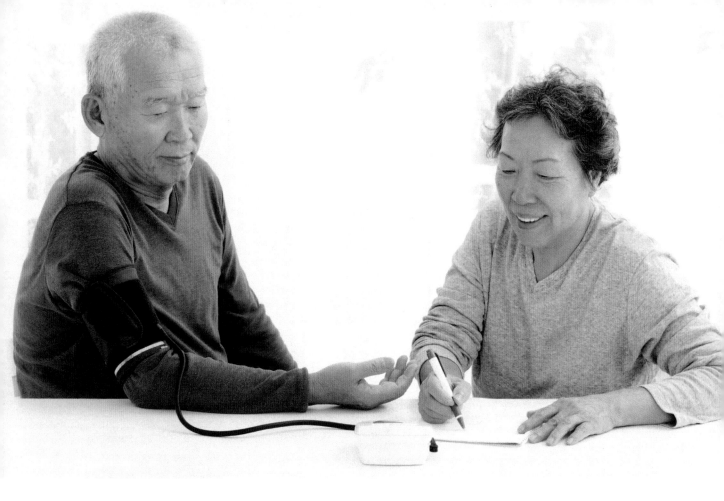

YOUR HEALTH BAG OF TRICKS

These tools can help you stay on top of your fitness, heart health and medication. Some are high-tech gizmos, while others are simple gadgets you may already own

BY JULIE STEWART

SOMETIMES, HAVING A SPECIAL tool to help get tasks done can make success easier, faster and more fun. With that in mind, we looked at 12 common health goals and found a great tool for each. Some are at the forefront of technology, but many are surprisingly simple, and might already be in your closet or kitchen drawer. Although you can manage your health issues yourself, these tips can give you a little boost—or provide a great service.

> **Monitor Your Fitness**
To reach your exercise goals faster, enlist a device that tracks your step count, distance logged and calories burned. A simple pedometer that handles those three measures can cost as little as $8; a more comprehensive tracker that feeds data to your phone or computer can run over $100. And if you want high style, designers are creating fashion-forward trackers and embellishments for the brands you already love.

> **Protect Your Skin**

Sunscreen is great, but it shouldn't be your only sun-shielding strategy. When you go out, don clothes woven, dyed or treated to block ultraviolet radiation. Look at the UPF, or Ultraviolet Protection Factor, number.

> **Keep Track of Heart Health**

Having blood pressure under 120/80 can help stave off a stroke. Check your numbers in the morning with a home blood pressure monitor. If you're already taking hypertension meds, a home monitor can help ensure your BP-lowering plan is working.

> **Measure Your Oxygen Levels**

A pulse oximeter passes light through your fingertip to measure the oxygen levels in your red blood cells. If you have chronic obstructive pulmonary disease (COPD), mention the device to your doc; it's not standard for COPD patients. Knowing your oxygen level can help you adjust your treatment.

> **Organize Your Pills**

The latest crop of automated pill organizers can be programmed to dispense exactly what you need at precisely the right time. They also can give alerts when it's medicine-taking time, and text a family member if you miss a dose.

> **Maintain Your Weight**

People who weigh themselves daily or even weekly are more likely to lose weight. The latest digital scales also send data to your phone, so you can catch upward trends before they balloon out of control.

> **Blend Your Nutrients**

If you need to get your nutrients in a hurry, drink them. Smoothies are delicious and nutritious (if you stick with ingredients like plain yogurt and fruits and vegetables). Your blender breaks down the fiber in food to make it easier to eat, while maintaining all the vitamins and minerals.

> **Care for Your Teeth**

Take your teeth to the next level with a power toothbrush, which can remove more plaque. Some models even include timers to help you brush your teeth for the full two to three minutes that most dental professionals recommend.

> **Relieve Chronic Pain**

TENS devices send tiny electrical pulses through aching tissue. TENS, or transcutaneous electrical nerve stimulation, can temporarily soothe back pain. Ask your doctor whether you're a candidate for an at-home TENS unit.

> **Soothe Muscle Soreness**

Foam rollers can help loosen your joints and reduce post-workout soreness, according to research from Canada. Roll over tender or tight spots with a soft polyethylene foam roller. Start with two to three sets of 15 seconds. Gradually increase by five to 10 seconds until you can do two to three sets of 60 seconds.

> **Protect Against Food Poisoning**

If you've ever eaten spoiled food, you know that nothing sends you on an all-out sprint to the restroom faster. Undercooked meats and poultry are common culprits in the home cook's kitchen, and cooking these items thoroughly can reduce your risk. But don't just eyeball it: Anything from the cut of the meat to the way it was packaged and stored could affect its color, according to a guide in *Meat Science*. To make sure your dinner is done, stick it with a meat thermometer, avoiding the bone (it will give you a false reading). Find the minimum safe temperatures here: http://www.foodsafety.gov/keep/charts/mintemp.html.

> **Stay Hydrated**

About 20 percent of otherwise healthy men and women participating in a study published in *Nutrients* turned out to be dehydrated. Today's smart bottles track your H_2O intake and tell you if you need to glug more, based on factors such as your age and exercise habits. ■

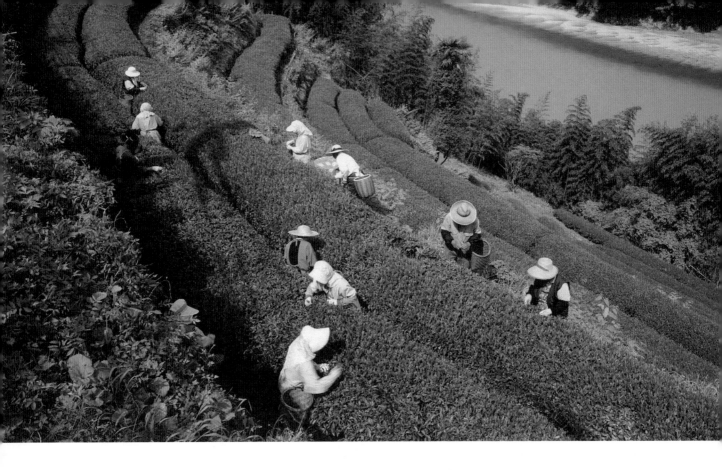

SECRETS FROM ONE OF THE LONGEST-LIVING PLACES ON EARTH

A healthy diet, among other things, contributes to a town's remarkable turnaround

BY KIRK SPITZER

TAKAMI KUROIWA LOOKS FOR-ward to weekends—not so he can relax with a little golf or TV, but to put in 12-hour days on the family farm. His regular job as a tourism manager provides a comfortable living, but raising his own fruit and vegetables is part of a lifelong routine. At 68, Kuroiwa has already come out of retirement once and expects to work well into his later years. "It's part of the lifestyle here. You work in an office and then you retire to the farm. It's just the next stage in life," Kuroiwa says. As it turns out, it's a very long life.

A healthy diet, regular physical activity, extended work years and aggressive government intervention have helped the Nagano region produce the longest life expectancy in Japan, which in turn is the longest in the world. That marks a remarkable turnaround for an area that, as recently as the early 1980s, had the highest rate of strokes in Japan.

> Challenges

At first glance, Nagano would seem an unlikely setting for a long and healthy life. Tucked high in the Japanese Alps, the area experiences long and harsh winters. Surrounded by mountains, Nagano is one of the few regions of Japan without immediate access to the fresh fish and seafood that makes up much of the national diet.

Even as Japan's economy boomed and longevity rates climbed through the postwar era, life expectancy in Nagano lagged. Men in particular suffered from high rates of stroke, heart attack and cerebral aneurysm. Much of the blame fell on a beloved, if unlikely, staple of the Nagano diet: pickled vegetables. One survey found that Nagano residents on average were consuming 15.1 grams of salt per day—by contrast, U.S. Dietary Guidelines urge people to eat no more than 2.3 grams a day.

> Focus on Diet

The first step in boosting Nagano's life span was a campaign to reduce salt consumption and promote a healthier diet and lifestyle. Miso soup, served three times a day in many homes, became a prime target of health officials. Cases of hypertension and related illnesses began to decline shortly after. The region of 2.1 million people now has some 4,750 volunteers who host seminars and clinics at supermarkets, shopping malls and community centers. They also conduct regular home visits to measure the salt content in daily meals and make dietary recommendations.

The efforts paid off with surprising speed. By 1990, life expectancy for men had risen three years in a decade in Nagano prefecture, and 3.5 years for women. Nagano life spans continued to climb until they topped all of Japan by 2010. Rates of deaths attributable to cancer, heart and liver disease, and pneumonia now rank well below the national average.

> Private Sector

As the effects of an improved diet began to be felt, the region's business community found ways to support a healthy lifestyle. In Matsumoto, the region's second largest city, a bank started offering higher interest rates and incentives like weekends at Tokyo's Disneyland for those who get medical checkups for three consecutive years.

City health workers will take blood pressure readings, answer questions and distribute information on public health care services. Those preventive care efforts contributed to lower health care costs in Nagano.

> Staying Active

Another not-so-secret key to Nagano's remarkable longevity is a vigorous lifestyle, encouraged by local leaders. Community groups and neighborhood associations organize communal walks—not difficult in group-oriented Japan. Even in winter, clusters of residents can be found regularly walking along Matsumoto's streets, parks and canals and around its historic medieval castle downtown.

Japanese officials encourage people to postpone retirement or begin second careers, in part to maintain a healthy lifestyle longer. Nagano is ahead of the curve there as well. Nearly 1 in 4 people over 65 are still in the workforce—the highest rate in Japan.

Kuroiwa says he doesn't think about all that. He retired as village accountant a few years ago, but came back to manage a new tourism center. As before, his spare time goes into running his family's small farm, where he grows apples and rice along with an array of vegetables. His parents worked regularly into their late 80s, and Kuroiwa figures he and his wife will do the same. ∎

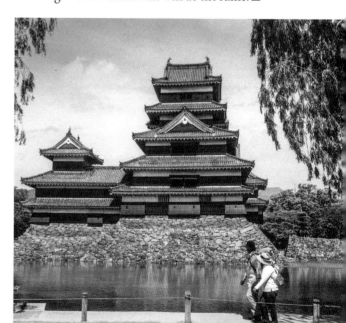

CREDITS

The 6 Rules for Eating Clean
by Jessica Levine, AARP The Magazine, April/May 2015

What to Expect in Your 50s, 60s, 70s and Beyond
by Beth Howard, AARP The Magazine, October 2012

Moves to Make You Healthier and Stronger
by Beth Howard, April 4, 2016

Get More Energy
by Sari Harrar, AARP.org

Increase Your Flexibility
AARP.org, August 31, 2016

Boost Your Bones at Any Age
by Amy Paturel, AARP The Magazine, February/March 2015

8 Ways to Prevent Arthritis
by Meghan Bogardus, updated July 2016

Normal Memory Problems
by Mary A. Fischer, AARP.org

Can Chess Help Your Brain?
by Renée Bacher, AARP.org

Boost Your Brain in 24 Hours
by Robin Westen, AARP.org

Tips for a Healthier Heart
by Jodi Helmer, July 25, 2015

Heart-Happy Foods with Omega-3 Oils
by Candy Sagon, June 29, 2016

High-Tech Heart Savers
by Amy Paturel, AARP The Magazine, February/March 2013

The Importance of Sleep
David Dudley, AARP The Magazine, August/September 2016

7 Daytime Habits to Help You Sleep Better
by Jessica Migala, March 18, 2016

Reset Your Body Clock for Better Brain Health
Michele Cohen Marill, August 25, 2016

Do You Really Need an Annual Physical?
by Candy Sagon, May 27, 2016

Your 50+ Vaccine Checklist
AARP.org

4 Surgeries You May Be Able to Avoid
by Karen Cheney, AARP The Magazine, August 2014

Getting the Nutrients You Need
by Amy Naturel, AARP The Magazine, January 14, 2015

Swallow with Care
by Elaine K. Howley, April 15, 2016

7 Ways to Ease Into Yoga
by Carol Krucoff, AARP Bulletin, January 14, 2011

Carol Krucoff, a yoga therapist at Duke Integrative Medicine in Durham, N.C., is codirector of the integrative yoga for seniors teacher training and the coauthor of Relax Into Yoga for Seniors.

Tai Chi May Boost Memory, Thinking Skills
by Janice Lloyd, AARP.org

The Meditation Cure
by Bill Stump, AARP The Magazine, April/May 2015

Your Health Bag of Tricks
by Julie Stewart, AARP.org

Secrets from One of the Longest-Living Places on Earth
by Kirk Spitzer, AARP Bulletin, May 2014

PHOTOGRAPHY CREDITS

A FINAL NOTE

It is often said that the body is the temple of the spirit. Although these words are ancient, they continue to resonate today. When we enter a house of worship, we tend to behave in a respectful, kind manner. If we care for our bodies with the same sort of reverence, we will be handsomely rewarded.

The message is not new: For better health, eat well, exercise, get enough rest, reduce stress, engage your mind, forge and maintain meaningful relationships. Although the advice is simple, the practice is not always easy, especially if we are not in the habit of following these guidelines. Don't be overwhelmed; instead, start where you are.

Begin by making small, gradual changes, such as eating lighter fare or taking a walk twice a week. As you become accustomed to your routine, deepen it by increasing your frequency and adding something new. If you're already swimming at the health club regularly, ask for a tour of the weight machines or try a yoga or Pilates class. If you've always eaten well but you're finding yourself lonely or with an abundance of time on your hands, stop by the local community center for an art class and some conversation. Don't look to renovate your temple in one day. Instead, embark on a journey to improve your health over time so you can live longer, better and healthier.

We get only one body in which to live our lives, and it's never too late to make changes for the better. Live well.

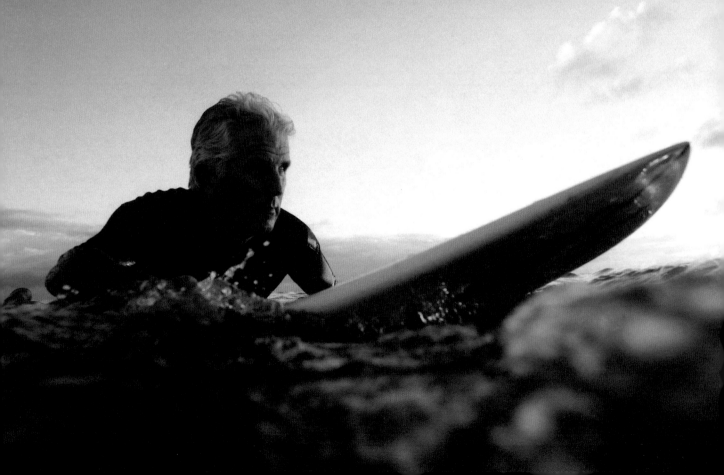

Made in the USA
Lexington, KY
10 March 2017